Case studies in neurological pain

This book is due for return on or before the last date shown below.

Case Studies in Neurological Pain

Claudia Sommer
Professor of Neurology at the University of Würzburg, Würzburg, Germany

Douglas W. Zochodne
Professor of Clinical Neurosciences at the Hotchkiss Brain Institute and the University of Calgary, Calgary, Alberta, Canada

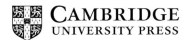
CAMBRIDGE
UNIVERSITY PRESS

CAMBRIDGE UNIVERSITY PRESS
Cambridge, New York, Melbourne, Madrid, Cape Town,
Singapore, São Paulo, Delhi, Mexico City

Cambridge University Press
The Edinburgh Building, Cambridge CB2 8RU, UK

Published in the United States of America by Cambridge
University Press, New York

www.cambridge.org
Information on this title: www.cambridge.org/9780521695268

First published 2012

Printed and bound in the United Kingdom by the MPG Books
Group

*A catalog record for this publication is available from the British
Library*

Library of Congress Cataloging in Publication data
Sommer, C. (Claudia)
Case studies in neurological pain / Claudia Sommer, Douglas
Zochodne.
    p.   ;   cm.
Includes bibliographical references and index.
ISBN 978-0-521-69526-8 (pbk.)
I. Zochodne, Douglas W.   II. Title.
[DNLM: 1. Neuralgia.   2. Nervous System Diseases –
complications. WL 544]
616.8 – dc23   2012020248

ISBN 978-0-521-69526-8 Paperback

Contents

Acknowledgments   vii

Introduction   1

Section A – The biology of neuropathic pain

1   **Mechanisms of neuropathic pain**   2

Section B – Focal, or localized neuropathies

2   **Pain and carpal tunnel syndrome**   16

3   **Pain and cervical radiculopathy**   19

4   **Pain and diabetic lumbosacral plexopathy**   23

5   **Pain and meralgia paresthetica**   27

6   **Pain and Lyme radiculopathy (borrelia-associated radiculitis)**   30

7   **Neuralgic amyotrophy**   34

8   **Painful radiculopathy associated with herpes zoster infection**   37

Section C – Generalized neuropathies or polyneuropathies

9   **Pain and chronic inflammatory demyelinating polyneuropathy**   41

10   **Pain and diabetic polyneuropathy (DPN)**   45

11   **Painful idiopathic polyneuropathy**   50

12   **Pain in vasculitic neuropathy**   54

13   **Painful polyneuropathy associated with anti-MAG autoantibodies**   59

14   **Painful polyneuropathy associated with inherited amyloidosis**   62

15   **Small fiber neuropathy in sarcoidosis**   66

16   **Pain and small fiber polyneuropathy in Fabry disease**   70

Section D – Other neuromuscular and neurological disorders

17   **Pain and proximal myotonic myopathy (DM2)**   74

18   **Complex regional pain syndrome**   77

19   **Pain and polymyalgia rheumatica**   82

20   **Phantom pain**   84

Section E – CNS disorders

21   **Pain in Parkinson's disease**   89

22   **Pain associated with amyotrophic lateral sclerosis (ALS)**   93

23   **Pain in Brown-Séquard syndrome**   96

24   **Pain in syringomyelia**   99

25   **Central pain with thalamic infarct**   104

26   **Pain in multiple sclerosis**   108

Section F – Headache disorders

27 **Chronic migraine**   113

28 **Cluster headache**   118

29 **Paroxysmal hemicrania**   122

30 **Trigeminal neuralgia**   126

31 **Headache and acute cerebral ischemia**   130

Section G – Treatment

32 **Therapeutics in neuropathic pain**   135

Index   138

Acknowledgments

Dr. Sommer acknowledges the help of Professor Lazlo Solymosi in providing radiological images and of Dr. José Perez for intraoperative photographs. Dr. Zochodne acknowledges the support of the Hotchkiss Brain Institute, University of Calgary and external funding from CIHR, CDA and AHFMR. Barbara Zochodne provided expert and detailed editorial assistance for drafts of the text. Sally Yakiwchuk provided citation proofing assistance. Jane Seakins of Cambridge Press provided ongoing publishing support and encouragement.

Introduction

Among all patients with neurological disorders, pain is probably the most common symptom experienced. Identifying, understanding, and treating pain is a responsibility of health care providers in all branches of neurology.

This text is about pain in neurological diseases, both "neuropathic" pain that is recognized in sensory neuron disorders but also other types of pain less commonly considered. These latter disorders include for example, pain in Parkinson's disease, ALS, and muscle diseases. The text includes specific chapters on mechanisms of neuropathic pain, updated with new ideas on its pathogenesis, and a summary of recent therapeutic guidelines. Most of the text however centers on actual patient encounters at the Neurology clinics of the Universities of Wurzburg and Calgary. This emphasis is to make the vignettes relevant to clinical practitioners but also to introduce researchers and workers in industry to the complex and challenging issues faced during direct patient encounters. Therapeutic failures are common among our vignettes, highlighting the fact that current therapeutic advances remain inadequate – a challenge for researchers to find better approaches.

In each section, we highlight a clinic patient case in a "vignette" emphasizing the patient's history, clinical findings, investigations, diagnosis, and treatment. Some vignettes indicate highly complex health care trajectories, another important lesson for non-clinicians. Despite the vignettes arising from widely separated health care environments in Canada and Germany, the similarities in these health care challenges are remarkable. Approximately half of the vignettes arise from each clinic. Keeping in mind that the literature is evolving and that some types of neurological pain have had limited attention, we review key literature points in each vignette and provide citations where possible. As might be expected, the citation density varies widely among these disorders indicating an uneven literature available to guide clinicians or instruct others. In many instances, illustrations are taken directly from the patients presented but other illustrations are also provided as general examples.

Medicine is a complex specialty that requires a tailored approach to care for individuals. While large cohorts of patients studied in clinical trials provide essential evidence on which to base practice, the reality is much more complex. We have hoped to convey these challenges, and some current insights into the associated neurological pain in this text.

Mechanisms of neuropathic pain

The clinical cases presented in this text highlight the variety of clinical neurological disorders associated with pain. As should be evident from the range of conditions presented and the parts of the nervous system they impact, pain can arise from any level of the neuraxis: sensory receptor to cortex. Similarly the disease processes that generate it are extensive from sensory neuropathies to thalamic cerebral infarction. The experience of pain is subjective, influenced by the context in which it occurs and the person in whom it develops. It may be painful to one person while it brings on a heightened, reduced or even absent response in another. The degree of pain is heavily influenced by the circumstances in which it occurs and the underlying psychological status of the sufferer. For example, patients with depression may have greater difficulty coping with pain and its intensity may be magnified by the concurrent problems they face. For these reasons, it is best described as a "pain experience," as distinguished from nociception, the transmission of potentially harmful stimuli through neuroanatomical "wiring" and neurochemical mediators.

"Neuropathic pain" is a subset of the pain experience specific to damage incurred in the nervous system. A current definition of neuropathic pain is provided by Treede and colleagues who describe it as "pain arising as a direct consequence of a lesion or disease affecting the somatosensory system" (1). In this description, neuropathic pain was graded on the following criteria: 1. pain with a distinct neuroanatomically plausible distribution; 2. a history suggestive of a relevent lesion or disease involving the peripheral or central somatosensory system; 3. demonstration of the distinct neuroanatomically plausible distribution by at least one confirmatory test; 4. demonstration of the relevant lesion or disease by at least one confirmatory test. With the above criteria, definite neuropathic pain met all 4, probable 1, 2 and 3 or 4, possible 1 and 2.

Strictly speaking, neuropathic pain has been used to refer to symptoms associated with neuropathy,

a disorder of the peripheral nervous system. Using this qualification, its characteristics share common descriptive features: burning, prickling, tingling (paresthesiae), electrical sensations, and pain generated by otherwise innocuous stimuli (allodynia). More recently, neuropathic pain has also been used to describe pain arising anywhere along the neuraxis. This broader usage has generated more descriptors, as demonstrated in the cases presented in this text.

This introductory chapter presents a brief overview of the mechanisms and mediators of pain in neurological conditions. It is a body of knowledge that is rapidly expanding beyond ideas that can be conveyed at the time of writing. Much of this knowledge has evolved from investigations of specific peripheral neuropathic pain mechanisms. The pain process involves the nervous system widely; even pain of exclusive peripheral origin may lead to secondary changes within the sensory ganglia, dorsal horn of spinal cord, brainstem, thalamus, and cortex. Major aspects are illustrated in a summary scheme [Figure 1.1]. We begin by discussing mechanisms that generate pain in the periphery at either damaged or intact distal axons and nerve terminals, and then proceed to analyze its development higher along the neuraxis.

Ectopic impulses

The development of the pain experience from distal injuries begins with ectopic, or unexpected spontaneous discharges from peripheral axons and their terminals. The terminals of axons that normally subserve nociception are found in the epidermis of the skin but also in many other tissues such as the meninges, liver capsule, joint capsule, periosteum, mesentery, and muscle. A large complement of afferent axons, usually unmyelinated "C" fibers, are normally found in nerves to muscles and serve to transmit painful stimuli. This explains why muscles can become painful after prolonged exercise or during needle electromyography.

MECHANISMS OF NEUROPATHIC PAIN

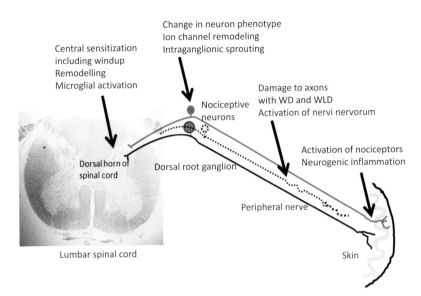

Change in neuron phenotype
Ion channel remodeling
Intraganglionic sprouting

Central sensitization
including windup
Remodelling
Microglial activation

Nociceptive
neurons

Damage to axons
with WD and WLD
Activation of nervi nervorum

Activation of nociceptors
Neurogenic inflammation

Dorsal horn of
spinal cord

Dorsal root ganglion

Peripheral nerve

Lumbar spinal cord

Skin

Figure 1.1. Simplified scheme identifying major events involving the neuraxis in the generation of neuropathic pain. These include (from right to left), activation of nociceptors with neurogenic inflammation, a cascade of molecular events associated with Wallerian (WD) and Wallerian-like degeneration (WLD) in the nerve trunk, alterations in neuronal phenotypes in the dorsal root ganglia with ion channel remodeling and intraganglionic sprouting, and changes in the dorsal horn of the spinal cord including remodeling, windup, and microglial activation.

At one time, it was also deliberately evoked by neurologists who tested patients for tabes dorsalis by identifying lack of sensation to deep pain while squeezing major proximal muscles. Tabes dorsalis, a tertiary complication of syphilis (neurosyphilis), inflames and damages the dorsal root entry zone of afferent fibers resulting in loss of deep pain sensitivity.

Normally nociception is transmitted by unmyelinated C axons and small myelinated Aδ axons with conduction velocities of 0.5–2.0 m/s and 12–30 m/s, respectively. It is not known whether specialized structures within these fibers are found at their terminals, but it is generally thought that they transmit nociception through "bare" or "free" nerve endings. They are stimulated by noxious mechanical, chemical, or thermal stimuli through specialized channels or receptors. A large complement of "silent" nociceptors, those only recruited during tissue damage and more significant injuries, may also exist.

In discussing neuropathic pain, our emphasis is on how damaged or diseased axons or neurons generate pain. Ectopic action potential discharges can be recorded from single axons proximal to a nerve trunk injury and their frequency has a strong direct correlation with the perceived intensity of pain. Ectopic discharges may be continuous or tonic, in phasic bursts, or completely irregular. How quiescent transmitting axons develop the capacity for generating ectopic

potentials is uncertain but the process likely involves a redistribution or alteration in their ion channels. Devor and colleagues demonstrated that injured axons swell to form axonal endbulbs, enlarged proximal portions of severed axons where axoplasmic material can accumulate (2). Within these endbulbs, accumulations of sodium channels, some inserted into the membrane, may be capable of generating ectopic activity. Specific blockers of these channels, such as phenytoin or lidocaine, interrupt spontaneous discharges. Several mechanisms are capable of changing the electrical properties of sodium channel subtypes Na_v 1.1 to 1.9 and thus the sensitivity of the respective nerve fiber (3, 4) [see below]. Genetic alterations in the sodium channel subtype Na_v 1.7 may lead to hyperactive channels. This is the pathophysiological basis of disorders such as erythromelalgia and paroxysmal extreme pain disorder (5). On the other hand, mutations that silence the channel lead to congenital insensitivity to pain (6).

In addition to structural alterations of individual damaged axons, pain may also arise from afferent fibers that self-innervate the peripheral nerve trunk. Nervi nervorum are unmyelinated axons found within the epineurial nerve sheath (7–9). This fascinating mechanism is considered in more detail later.

The activation or sensitization of peripheral axons, especially after injury, involves the participation of a range of pain-generating and pain-attenuating molecules, considered below. The sheer numbers of players involved has prompted diverse thoughts on therapy and intervention to treat neuropathic pain.

Algesic molecules

Within the vicinity of an injured peripheral nerve axon, a range of newly expressed molecules are capable of facilitating ectopic discharges that result in pain. These molecules are termed algesic. Extracellular potassium, released from dead and dying cells, helps to depolarize nearby axons. Similarly, there may be accumulation of hydrogen ions in ischemic acidotic injured tissues that activate acid-sensitive ion channels and TRP channels (see below). Several algesic molecules likely influence the excitability of damaged axons by synergistic interactions, or by changing the properties of the final common pathway mediated by ion channels expressed on axons. Specific ion channels are described below.

Combinations of algesic molecules released from local macrophages and leukocytes comprise an "inflammatory soup" that generates neuropathic pain: these include tumour necrosis factor α (TNFα), nitric oxide (NO), interleukin-1β (IL-1β), proteases that act on PAR2 receptors, and others. Algesic molecules are linked with generating pain behavior in experimental animal models. Histamine is associated with the development of closely related sensory symptoms including both pain and itch. Nerve growth factor (NGF) is a potent algesic substance causing sensations of deep aching pain when injected subcutaneously or intramuscularly. NGF may act through its high affinity TrkA receptors, known to be expressed in small caliber sensory axons that subserve nociception.

Neuropeptides, such as substance P (SP) and calcitonin gene-related peptide (CGRP), are released by sensory axons in tissues during injury. It is possible that they auto-reactivate the sensory axons that originally released them to amplify pain sensations. Better described however, is a pathway in which SP and CGRP act on mast cells to release histamine and serotonin as direct algesic molecules. Bradykinin is an algesic molecule that arises from the proteolytic cleavage product of kininogen during inflammation. Bradykinin acts on B1 and B2 receptors, both of which are upregulated in sensory ganglia after a peripheral injury. B2 receptors rise early, within 48 h of injury, whereas B1 receptors rise later, by 14 days. Both contribute toward pain behavior as demonstrated by phar-

macological inhibitors to either bradykinin receptor that dampen neuropathic pain in rats (10).

ATP acts as an algesic molecule through specific purinergic receptors that include P2X3, P2X2/3, P2X4, P2X7, and P2Y. Alternatively, P2X3 antagonists are analgesic. P2X receptors are nonselective cation channels permeable to calcium, sodium, and potassium with downstream actions on the MAPK pathway. Whereas P2X3, P2X2/3, and P2Y activate neurons directly, P2X4 and P2Y may activate neurons indirectly through the activation of nearby microglia (11). P2Y may also modulate TRPV1 receptors and increase their sensitivity (see below). In a related pathway, P1 receptors activated by adenosine inhibit nociception.

During peripheral nerve injury, there is rapid expression of inflammatory mediators produced by intrinsic cells such as Schwann cells, endothelial cells, and fibroblasts in the early phase, within hours. These mediators are also expressed by invading macrophages and T-lymphocytes at later phases over several days. One interesting scenario involves a sequence of events that follows initial primary axon damage: activation of Schwann cells occurs as a result of calcium released from damaged axons (12), the activation of Toll-like receptors (13), and the subsequent production of pro-inflammatory cytokines, chemokines. Additional molecules involved in this process include calpain (14, 15) and later glutamate (16). Chemokines such as CCL-2, in addition to their release by inflammatory cells, may be packed into neuronal synaptic vesicles and serve as neurotransmitters in the spinal cord (17, 18). After injury, Schwann cells and hematogenous macrophages newly express iNOS (inducible nitric oxide synthase), a potent generator of NO, an additional inflammatory mediator (19).

Prostaglandins synthesized by cyclooxygenases (COX1 and COX2), especially PGE2, are also mediators of pain during inflammation. COX2 may be the more important of the two cyclooxygenase enzymes during neuropathic pain and it is mainly expressed by Schwann cells and inflammatory cells such as macrophages after nerve injury (20–22). PGE2 acting through its EP1 receptors activates sodium and potassium channels in neurons, inhibits potassium channels, releases SP and CGRP, and sensitizes neurons to bradykinin and capsaicin (23).

Proteinase-activated receptors (PARs) are a special class of cell surface receptors activated by proteinases such as thrombin, trypsin, mast cell tryptase, and others (24). Cleavage at their extracellular amino terminus exposes a tethered ligand that in turn activates the receptor. PAR1 and PAR2 are expressed on sensory afferents, and PAR2 agonists can induce the release of SP and CGRP by sensory neurons to promote hyperalgesia (25). In contrast, PAR1 agonists are associated with analgesia (26).

Taken together, it is highly likely that the neuropathic phenotype arises from a combination of algesic molecules, in turn overcoming endogenous forms of analgesia, considered next.

Analgesic molecules

Injured peripheral nerves also express analgesic mediators that dampen pain sensations. The endogenous opioids are the most prominent. For example, β endorphin and met-enkephalin are expressed by inflammatory cells at injury sites (27, 28). This form of expression may attenuate pain by altering the release of algesic molecules from inflammatory cells that infiltrate the injured nerve. In addition however, endogenous opioids can act directly on local μ opioid receptors expressed by axons, including axonal endbulbs. For example, ligation of μ opioid receptors by small near nerve doses of agonists reversed features of experimental neuropathic pain including thermal hyperalgesia and mechanical allodynia (29).

Nociceptin (orphanin FQ) is an analgesic molecule that acts on opioid receptor-like 1 (ORL1) receptors. Both the ligand and receptor are expressed by DRG sensory neurons and their expression increases following peripheral inflammatory stimuli (30). Part of their analgesic action arises from suppression of inflammatory pain mediators.

Cannabinoids are analogs of Δ^9-tetrahydrocannabinol (THC), the active ingredient of marijuana. They operate as analgesics by acting on two separate receptors, labeled CB1 and CB2 (31–33). CB1 receptors are found in the central and peripheral nervous system where they inhibit calcium influx and enhance inward-rectifying potassium channels. In contrast, CB2 receptors are largely localized to immune cells (mast cells, T cells, B cells, NK cells, microglial cells, and macrophages in addition to monocytes and PMNs) and keratinocytes. Expression may also be found on microglial cells in the dorsal horn of the spinal cord that are activated following nerve injury. After nerve injury CB2 receptor expression is dramatically upregulated on primary sensory neurons. Thus, inhibition of CB1 receptors, CB2 receptors or both

attenuate neuropathic pain but CB1 inhibition may cause undesirable side-effects because of its unrelated actions on neurons (31).

Anti-inflammatory cytokines such as IL-4 and IL-10 not only counteract pro-inflammatory cytokines but also appear to have an intrinsic analgesic action (34). Overall, these molecules are coordinated within an anti-inflammatory systemic cytokine profile that attenuates neuropathic pain in humans with peripheral neuropathy (35).

Galanin is a neuropeptide that can influence pain behavior. Activation of its GALR1 receptors inhibits nociception, whereas its GALR2 receptors are excitatory. By blocking SP and CGRP action and increasing the actions of morphine, its predominant action during peripheral nerve injury or inflammation is analgesic (36). Finally, the neurotrophic molecule NT-3 acts to reduce thermal hyperalgesia by downregulating the expression of TRPV1 channels (see below) (37).

We next consider how specific anatomical sites of the peripheral nervous system and spinal cord participate in the generation of neuropathic pain. We start by considering how axons participate in peripheral inflammation.

Neurogenic inflammation and nervi nervorum

Tissue damage that generates pain is closely associated with *neurogenic inflammation*. Neurogenic inflammation refers to the active participation of terminal sensory axons in expanding and intensifying an inflammatory reaction associated with tissue damage. Classically, activated sensory axons within inflamed tissues send discharges back toward the central nervous system. At branch points along the activated sensory axon tree, axons arising send backfired antidromic (the reverse direction of physiological axon activation) discharges down axons where they release neuropeptides (38, 39). Because these territories are adjacent to those originally associated with sensory terminal activation (branch territories), the release of these neuropeptides can thereby enlarge the inflammatory response. SP and CGRP are potent vasodilators, whereas SP also causes plasma extravasation from vessels. Both may act on mast cells, causing their degranulation and release of histamine, serotonin, and proteases (39).

Through neurogenic inflammation, local neuropeptides contribute to the cardinal signs of inflammation in tissues, as elegantly described by Lewis

(38, 40): dolor (pain), rubor (redness from rises in blood flow), and tumor (swelling from plasma extravasation). Peripheral nerve trunks, self-innervated by SP and CGRP nervi nervorum axons in their epineurial sheaths, also undergo this type of enhanced inflammation (7). It is possible that inflammatory neuropathies may generate neuropathic pain through this mechanism without the presence of overt axon damage (8, 9).

Overactive neurogenic inflammation may also contribute to pain syndromes such as complex regional pain syndromes I and II (CRPS I and II). CRPS I by definition does not include actual nerve damage, whereas CRPS II does. Reflex sympathetic dystrophy (RSD) is a term previously applied to CRPS; adrenergic overactivity was thought to be involved in its pathogenesis. The evidence for prominent adrenergic involvement however, has been limited and other mechanisms may account for its features. For example, chronic activation of SP and CGRP containing C nociceptors may better account for the redness and swelling that accompany CRPS (41, 42). Next we discuss how axon degeneration may generate inflammation and pain.

Inflammation, Wallerian degeneration, Wallerian-like degeneration

Following nerve injury, axons and neurons are exposed to inflammatory pain mediators, or algesic molecules as discussed above. Specific inflammatory disorders of peripheral nerves, such as vasculitis, CIDP or GBS, may be expected to attract large numbers of lymphocytes and macrophages to the endoneurium. After simple axon injuries however, such as transection or crush, an inflammatory cascade also occurs. Augustus Waller described a sequence of pathological changes that develop distal to sharp nerve transections since referred to as Wallerian degeneration (WD) (43). Wallerian-like degeneration (WLD) refers to a near identical sequence of events in distal axons that may follow a crush or occur in other neuropathies.

Within 1–2 days following injury, axonal swellings or endbulbs develop in proximal stump axons. Their potential role in elaborating neuropeptides and expressing sodium channels was considered above. Later, by days 3–5 following nerve injury, there is an influx of macrophages into the injured peripheral nerve that is accompanied by cytokines, chemokines, NGF, NO, and other molecules. Previous studies have outlined the timetable of cytokine and chemokine expression during WD with both early rises in some mediators and later rises in others. One working hypothesis suggests that neuropathic pain may be triggered and maintained as a function of the intensity of the nearby inflammatory milieu. In conditions such as diabetes, where the onset and clearance of inflammation is delayed, neuropathic pain may be prolonged (44). During regeneration and clearance of the products of WD, neuropathic pain diminishes. The only caveat to this concept is that regenerating sprouts can exhibit mechanosensitivity and may promote some types of neuropathic pain during recovery.

Next we discuss how DRG sensory neurons participate in pain generation.

Changes within sensory dorsal root ganglia and their terminals

Sensory dorsal root ganglia (DRGs) that house the cell bodies, or perikarya, of sensory neurons, participate in the development of neuropathic pain. Normally, DRG neurons can be segregated into various types depending on their size, peptide content, and other properties (45). Small sensory neurons are classically associated with nociception, express SP, CGRP, and also express TrkA receptors that are ligated by NGF. A second population of small sensory neurons are known as non-peptidergic, are responsive to GDNF, express the GDNF and neurturin receptors GFRα1 and GFRα2, respectively, and have a binding site for the *Griffonia simplicifolia* IB4 plant lectin. These neurons project to lamina IIi (inner portion of lamina II) and are referred to as NGF unresponsive small afferents. Thus, these neurons differ from TrkA neurons that project to laminae I and IIo. After axon injuries, DRG neurons change their phenotype in numerous ways, facilitating pain discharges and allowing them to act as independent generators of ectopic discharges. Thus, after a peripheral axon lesion, ectopic discharges can arise not only from damaged axons at the injury site, but also from their parent DRG neurons. DRG neurons assume pacemaker-like properties, generating spontaneous ectopic discharges that correlate with pain intensity (2).

The alterations in DRG neurons associated with axon injury and neuropathic pain involve expression of specific ion channel subtypes. Both rises and declines in specific channels have been described: declines in Na_v 1.9 (NaN/SNS2; TTX resistant, found in small to medium sized neurons), Na_v 1.8 (SNS/PN3; TTX resistant; found in small neurons), I_{KIR} (inwardly rectifying), and K_v1.4 (fast transient potassium channel, small neurons) and rises in Na_v1.3 (sodium channel, Naβ3 subunit in small neurons) and KCNQ2,3,5 (related to potassium channels and associated with M currents). Still other changes are described in large DRG sensory neurons but their association with neuropathic pain is uncertain, e.g., declines in K_v 1.1,1.2, T Ca^{2+}, K_vβ2.1, and I_{KIR}. Some ion channel changes in both large and small neurons differ when the ganglia are inflamed or exposed to NGF (see review by Lawson (46)).

Alterations in Na_v1.7 (PN1 or hNE9), also expressed in DRG sensory neurons, are of considerable interest (47). For example, lack of functional Na_v1.7 is associated with insensitivity to pain but paradoxically a pain syndrome known as erythromelalgia can arise from mutations of Na_v1.7. The mutated channel has altered properties that promote hyperexcitability of neurons. Patients with erythromelalgia describe the cardinal features of neuropathic pain including chronic burning sensations of the limbs. An additional pain syndrome known as paroxysmal extreme pain disorder (PEPD) is associated with a separate distinct mutation of Na_v1.7. Unexpected expression of Na_v1.7 has been identified in the axons of chronic human neuromas where they may contribute toward ectopic discharges and neuropathic pain (48). Recently, Faber et al. (49) identified missense gain of function mutations of Na_v1.7 that result in neuronal hyperexcitability in 8 of 28 patients with idiopathic painful small fiber neuropathy. The collaboration with Na_v1.8, nearly exclusively expressed in DRG sensory neurons, is also involved in the pain syndromes linked to mutant Na_v1.7 channels. Na_v1.8 may also be a critical player in other types of neuropathic pain (47). The hyperpolarization-activated, cyclic nucleotide-gated cation channel (HCN2) in Na_v1.8 expressing nociceptors appears to be critical for the firing of these neurons after nerve injury and in inflammation (50). The roles of Na_v1.9 and Na_v1.3 are less clear.

Sensory neurons also express A-type K+ channels that attenuate pain. Two subtypes known as Kv3.4 and Kv4.3 have distinguished themselves; when these subtypes are suppressed by antisense oligodeoxynucleotides, rats develop mechanical hyperalgesia without thermal hyperalgesia (51).

There are changes in calcium channel expression and function, including their interaction with adrenergic receptors (52, 53) after axon injury. A notable example is the α2δ-1 calcium channel subunit, upregulated after axon injury, and now known to be the target of the analgesic compounds pregabalin and gabapentin (54–56). N-type calcium channels (Ca_v2.2) may be particularly important in the generation of neuropathic and chronic pain. Widely distributed in the nervous system, these channels exhibit high density expression in DRG neurons and in the synaptic terminals of the dorsal horn, laminae I and II. In the dorsal horn of the spinal cord, N-type channels control glutamate and SP release (57). Peptides isolated from cone snails, such as ω-conotoxin-MVIIA and ω-conotoxin-GVIA that block N-type calcium channels, are potent analgesic molecules (58, 59). Moreover, there are two calcium channel splice isoforms of N-type calcium channels labeled e37a and e37b that have differing properties (60). E37a is expressed in 55% of nociceptive capsaicin-sensitive neurons, and contributes to SP release. E37a knockdown blocks basal thermal and mechanical nociception, thermal and mechanical inflammatory hyperalgesia tested using the formalin paw test, and thermal hyperalgesia in the chronic constriction (CCI) neuropathic pain model. E37b has fewer effects overall but alters tactile allodynia. Inhibition of the binding of collapsin response mediator protein 2 (CRMP-2) to Ca_v2.2 decreased neuropeptide release from DRG neurons and reduced excitatory synaptic transmission in the spinal cord dorsal horn (61).

In addition to ion channels, there is a wide repertoire of molecular changes in DRG sensory neurons that have sustained an injury to their axons. Some are associated with the development of pain, whereas others prepare neurons for regenerative activity (RAGs, or regeneration associated genes). Morphological changes accompany alterations of RAGs, retrograde changes known as the "cell body reaction" (or the "axon reaction": central chromatolysis and displacement of nuclei to the periphery of the cell (62)). Medium diameter sensory afferents, newly expressing SP, initiate the transmission of pain information. After axotomy, small neurons upregulate galanin, a potential analgesic peptide, downregulate μ opioid receptors, and downregulate the peptides SP and CGRP, the TrkA NGF receptor, and P2X3 purinergic receptors. P2X3 receptors are prominent on IB4 non-peptidergic neurons. After injury, large neurons upregulate BDNF,

TNFα, NPY, and α2 adrenergic receptors. In contrast to the downregulation of opioid receptors after injury described above, a partial nerve injury model showed increases in μ-opioid receptors (MORs) expressed by sensory neurons ipsilateral to the injury (29). Peripheral inflammation also generates rises in CGRP, SP, and BDNF in DRG neurons that contrast to the declines observed after injury (63).

DRG neurons express κ and δ opioid receptors, sometimes colocalized, that influence pain transmission and that may change during inflammation (64). Small DRG neurons express δ-opioid receptors (DOR) that, like MORs, are analgesic (63). Nociceptin and its receptor ORL1 are expressed in larger numbers of DRG neurons after peripheral inflammatory lesions (30).

Sensory neurons that are not primarily injured but housed in the same DRG as injured neighbors may change their phenotype in ways that promote neuropathic pain. This interesting phenomenon may arise from interactions of intact "en passant" axons with inflammatory mediators associated with damaged neighbours, or through interactions within the DRG itself. Examples of neurons that change their DRG phenotype when not directly injured are those containing CGRP (65) and P2X3 (66). P2X3 receptors, discussed above, are cation channels activated by ATP, exclusively localized to DRG and trigeminal sensory neurons. They may facilitate pain neurotransmission. CGRP, as discussed above, arises from small and medium sized sensory neurons. It has a role in neurogenic inflammation as a vasodilator and potentiates SP nociceptive signaling in the dorsal horn of the spinal cord.

Another important family of molecules expressed by sensory neurons are the transient receptor potential proteins (TRPs), ion channels permeable to cations. The classical TRP channels include the capsaicin receptor (TRPV1) that mediates heat and acid stimuli and the TRPM8 or menthol channel that mediates cold sensations. Other TRPs include TRPV2,3,4 and TRPA1 (mild warming for TRPV4; moderate warming to 31°C for TRPV3, heat for TRPV1 and noxious heat for TRPV2 with mild cooling by TRPM8 and noxious cooling by TRPA1). Ipsilateral to a partial nerve injury (CCI, chronic constriction injury), increases in TRPA1, TRPV1, TRPV2, and TRPM8 were observed (37, 67). Rises in TRPV1 occur in small to medium sized neurons in the DRG and could be suppressed by NT-3 (37). TRPM8 (transient receptor potential

melastatin 8), the cold- and menthol-sensitive receptor neurons comprise 5–10% of the DRG neuron population; this proportion increased ipsilateral to an experimental neuropathic lesion (chronic constriction injury) along with a rise in their sensitivity (68). This may be a mechanism for the process of cold allodynia, the perception of innocuous cold stimuli as painful.

Acid-sensing ion channels (ASICs) also participate in the generation of pain, with functions and expression patterns that overlap with TRPs (69). These are voltage-independent depolarizing cation channels largely used by sodium ions. The PNS expresses ASIC 1a,b, 2a,b, and ASIC3. ASIC3 are the most well characterized and serve as mediators of acid-induced cutaneous pain, integrators of thermal hypersensitivity during inflammation, and mediators of muscle pain. Bohlen et al. (70) examined the toxin from the venom of the Texus coral snake (*Micrurus tener tener*) and purified a toxin responsible for the intense pain generated by this venom. The toxin, MitTx, was highly selective for ASIC1a and 1b channels.

In addition to morphological and molecular changes in parent neuron perikarya after injury, there are also changes in the behavior of their neighbouring glial cells. Sensory neurons in DRG are closely surrounded by perineuronal satellite cells, cytoplasmic poor relatives of SCs that closely wrap them. Remarkably, these cells enlarge and proliferate after injury indicating a sensitivity to events involving the neuron some distance away. While it is known that satellite cells can elaborate growth factors, it is also possible that they participate in the neuronal remodeling that leads to neuropathic pain. This hypothesis remains unexplored. Macrophages influx into DRG after distal axotomy and can elaborate IL-6, and likely other inflammatory mediators (71–74). Thus, both changes in perikaryal properties and involvement in neighboring cells may allow DRGs to act as pacemakers as neuropathic pain develops.

Injuries to peripheral nerves also induce retrograde sprouting of sympathetic adrenergic axons from nearby perivascular innervation into ganglia (75–77). The axons form pericellular basket-like structures in which tyrosine hydroxylase (TH) varicosities contact sensory neuron perikarya. This interesting property depends on NGF availability in the ganglia as a result of retrograde transport of the growth factor from target tissues. Noradrenergic sympathetic sprouting varies in its latency of onset in experimental nerve injury and pain models. This intriguing phenomenon may be related to "sympathetically mediated pain" as described in CRPS I and II (Chapter 18).

The possibility that neuropathic pain might also be generated by direct damage to DRGs is also a consideration. Relatively little work has examined the consequences of direct traumatic DRG injury. The possibility that common pain syndromes such as cervical or lumbar spondylosis may involve compression and damage of DRG neurons is addressed in Chapter 3 (cervical radiculopathy).

Alterations in DRG neuronal behavior "feed forward" into altered processing of pain discharges in the central nervous system, considered next.

Role of the dorsal horn of spinal cord

The dorsal horn of the spinal cord (and the nucleus of the spinal trigeminal tract) is the first central afferent center to receive nociceptive discharges. Their complex circuitry predictably influences the information that ascends to other CNS centers. Similarly, their output can be modified by descending systems that are largely anti-nociceptive but also pro-nociceptive. As one might expect, their connections also undergo important changes in the setting of peripheral nerve injury or inflammation.

The dorsal horn is divided into Rexed laminae, the outermost of which by definition is layer I. Unmyelinated C afferents largely synapse in layer II (IB4 neurons may also synapse in layer I), also known as the substantia gelatinosa. Small myelinated Aδ nociceptive afferents synapse in layers I and V. The most important neurotransmitter released by afferents is glutamate, in turn acting on NMDA and AMPA receptors of second order sensory fibers or interneurons (63). Other neurotransmitters that act in concert with glutamate include the neuropeptides SP and CGRP. Dorsal horn neurons can be classified as projection neurons with axons travelling to higher centers or interneurons that are capable of influencing pain transmission. The projection neurons are more likely to be found in lamina I and they cross the midline to ascend in the spinothalamic tract (78). Interneurons are classified as nociceptive-specific (majority), polymodal, or wide dynamic range, coding both innocuous and injurious stimuli and they synapse, among others, with projection neurons. Many interneurons also demonstrate the property of windup referring to an increase in their sensitivity with repeated stimuli. This property is mediated by glutamate through NMDA (N-methyl-D-

aspartate) receptors. Predictably, infusion of NMDA intrathecally in rats generates a regional pain syndrome (79). Recently, zinc has been discovered to be an endogenous modulator of excitatory neurotransmission in the spinal cord through NMDA receptors containing a particular subunit named NR2A (80). The adipocytokine leptin is a molecule that enhances NMDA receptor function in neuropathic pain (81, 82).

Mapping the activation of the proto-oncogene c-fos protein Fos has allowed analysis of the neuroanatomic basis of pain pathway participation after injury or inflammation, and its modulation (e.g., by analgesics) (see review by Coggeshall (83)). Fos rapidly rises in neurons during activation of the nociceptive or pain pathways and its behavior is specific, induced by few stimuli beyond pain. Although its expression can persist in chronic pain states, its expression is typically short-term in a maximum range of 30 min to 2 h. This facilitates its analysis in acute pain studies. Laminae I and II develop intense expression of Fos after noxious stimuli followed by upregulation in lamina V and others. Higher centers that express Fos include the reticular formation, the nucleus of the solitary tract, the parabrachial nucleus, the periaqueductal gray, the locus coeruleus, the hypothalamus, the thalamus, and the cortex. Fos upregulation follows peripheral nerve lesions, spinal cord damage, dorsal root avulsion, and DRG irritation. Interestingly, simple dorsal root injury does not activate Fos. As expected from the earlier discussion, Fos expression can be attenuated by a range of analgesics including: opioids, NMDA antagonists, GABA$_B$ agonists, NK1 antagonists, cannabinoids, and nonsteroidal anti-inflammatory agents (83).

The remodeling of architecture in the dorsal horn of the spinal cord following nerve injury is not confined to neurons. Microglia, described as the resident inflammatory cells of the CNS, are activated in the dorsal horn within 24 h of a peripheral nerve injury. There are morphological changes, proliferation, and rises in expression of several critical molecules including CR3, toll-like receptor-4, CD14, CD4, and MC class II protein (84). Key microglial proteins such as P2X4 receptors and the second messenger p38 MAP kinase are likely critical in mediating pain signals. Microglia may facilitate pain signaling by dampening dorsal horn inhibitory mechanisms or facilitating excitation. BDNF released from microglia appears to be an important participant in central sensitization (85). Beggs and Salter (86) suggest that enhanced BDNF release acts on lamina I neurons of the doral horn

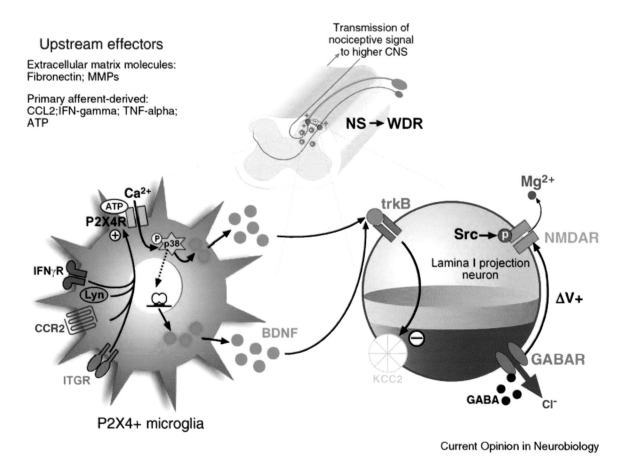

Upstream effectors

Extracellular matrix molecules:
Fibronectin; MMPs

Primary afferent-derived:
CCL2;IFN-gamma; TNF-alpha;
ATP

Current Opinion in Neurobiology

Figure 1.2. Hypothesis linking events in microglia with projection neurons in the dorsal horn of the spinal cord as proposed by Beggs and Salter (86). In this scheme, activation of P2X4 receptors increases BDNF synthesis and release through a p38MAPK-dependent mechanism. BDNF downregulates KCC2 channels in the membranes of dorsal horn lamina I neurons, reducing GABA inhibition and increasing neuronal excitability in response to NMDA receptor agonists. The overall result is to change neurons that are normally nociceptive-specific to become wide dynamic range in phenotype, increasing hyperalgesia, allodynia, and spontaneous pain. Reproduced with permission from Beggs and Salter (86).

through TrkB receptors to suppress KCC2 chloride transporters. This increases intraneuronal Cl⁻ levels, leading to a role of GABA receptors in rendering neuron hyperexcitability. Both diminished GABA inhibition and facilitated glutamatergic input contribute to a change in neurons from a nociceptive specific to wide dynamic range phenotype, contributing to hyperalgesia, allodynia, and spontaneous pain [Figure 1.2].

Diminished synaptic inhibition may also be caused by spinal endocannabinoids using CB1 receptors, which are activated upon strong nociceptive simulation and reduce the release of GABA and glycine (87). Overall, changes in the excitability of the dorsal horn involve several mechanisms that include specific changes in spontaneous excitability (88), windup

enhancement of central sensitivity through NMDA (89, 90), and loss of GABAergic inhibition (91).

Brainstem relays and the descending modulation of pain

There are two main brainstem pain centers: the parabrachial area found in the midbrain and rostral pons and the periaqueductal gray area of the midbrain. Parabrachial neurons project to the amygdala and ventrolateral and medial hypothalamus (78). The periaqueductal gray area projects descending axons to the spinal cord. Closely associated with the periaqueductal gray neurons are those of the rostral ventromedial medulla.

Descending input into the dorsal horn of the spinal cord arises from several neuroanatomical loci (92). Monosynaptic inputs into the dorsal horn arise from the hypothalamus, the parabrachial nucleus, the nucleus tractus solitarius, the brainstem nucleus raphe magnus, the rostroventromedial medulla, the dorsal reticular nucleus, the cerebral cortex, and the periaqueductal gray area in the midbrain. Several neurotransmitters are involved. Norepinephrine inhibits primary afferents and projection neurons directly and inhibits projection neurons indirectly through enkephalin and GABA interneurons. Similar inhibitory pathways use dopamine and serotonin. Serotonin acts on $5HT_3$ receptors expressed on interneurons, but probably also on $5\text{-}HT_2$ receptors on interneurons, $5\text{-}HT_{1A}$ receptors on projection neurons and $5\text{-}HT_{1B/D}$ receptors on primary afferents. Both serotonin and norepinephrine, the latter released from axons arising in the locus coeruleus, dampen nociceptive afferent discharges.

Treatment of pain using spinal cord stimulation is based on activation of the descending analgesic system. Descending pathways can include facilitatory circuits, also mediated by norepinephrine, dopamine, and serotonin (92).

Thalamic participation in pain

Nociceptive input into the thalamus is divided into the lateral sensory-discriminative and medial motivational-affective systems (93). The lateral input constitutes the ventral posterior nucleus of the thalamus. The medial nuclei include the intralaminar (centromedian, centrolateral, and parafascicular) and midline nuclei. The lateral nuclei have better facility to identify the location and intensity of pain and they project to the somatosensory cortex. The medial nuclei project to the anterior cingulate gyrus.

Cortical pain centers

The participation of the CNS in pain perception was comprehensively reviewed by Hudson (93). Several parts of the human cerebrum participate in pain perception. One of the most important is the cingulate gyrus, a part of the limbic system found above and along the corpus callosum. The cingulate cortex contains opioid receptors, and receives projections from midline and intralaminar nuclei of the thalamus. The

rostral anterior cingulate gyrus (including Brodmann area 24) likely contributes to emotional responses during pain. The anterior cingulate has close reciprocal connections to its posterior counterpart which, in turn, connects to the parietal cortex, occipital cortex, striatal nuclei, and thalamic nuclei. Other cortical areas that participate in pain responses include the parietal somatosensory areas (S1, and S2 or Brodmann areas 3, 1, 2) and the insula which in turn is closely connected to the somatosensory cortex and the amygdala. The insula is also thought to participate in affective components of the pain experience.

The prefrontal cortex (especially area 10) may integrate inputs through reciprocal connections to the somatosensory cortex and the anterior cingulate gyrus. Patients who previously underwent prefrontal leucotomy for intractable pain reported loss of the unpleasant aspect of their pain experience. All of these cortical areas naturally have widespread connections elsewhere including the motor cortices and basal ganglia. These may become activated (as detected on PET and fMRI studies) during painful states. Furthermore, these sites in turn may elicit motor responses through their connections to the motor outputs. Surprisingly, the amygdala, associated with emotional behavior, and the hippocampus, associated with memory formation, may be inactive during pain states. Nonetheless, the amygdala is connected to the periaqueductal grey nucleus of the brainstem that in turn, is very much activated during pain. The amygdala is also connected to the hypothalamus that is involved in the autonomic responses to painful stimuli.

Recent insights into the participation and plasticity of the anterior cingulate cortex (gyrus; ACC) are provided by Zhuo (94). Painful inputs into the ACC as well as forebrain and insular cortex trigger unpleasant sensations and experiences. The somatosensory cortex, in contrast, is thought to help determine the location and quality of pain, whereas the hippocampus may contribute to pain-related spatial memory. Electrophysiological recordings from ACC neurons have identified responses to injury and specific nociceptor neurons. Plastic properties observed within ACC neurons have included long-term potentiation and depression, mediated through alterations in glutamate receptor signaling, NMDA (N-methyl-D-aspartate) receptors, and calcium-calmodulin activated adenylyl cyclases (94). All of these properties have highlighted parallel forms of neuronal behavior in pain and memory.

11

Summary

Neuropathic pain involves a complex and redundant system of wiring and molecules that is only slowly being unraveled. While initial pain generators are found in target tissues and in the primary afferent sensory axons that innervate them, the "pain experience," if prolonged, involves multiple levels of the neuraxis. When the "wiring" is primarily damaged in neurological disease, a level of further complexity is added that contributes toward the amplification and persistence of pain. The neuroanatomical changes involve a combination of dorsal and higher circuit remodeling, recruitment of microglia, inappropriate sprouting of axons within DRGs, and reparative changes in the distal axons. The molecular changes are diverse and include changes in both pro- and antinociceptive systems. Prominent among these are alterations in ion channel properties of neurons; upregulation of cytokines, chemokines, and inflammatory peptides; changes in the expression of opioids and cannabinoids; altered TRP channels; and changes in NMDA receptors.

References

(1) Treede RD, Jensen TS, Campbell JN, et al. Neuropathic pain: redefinition and a grading system for clinical and research purposes. *Neurology* 2008;70:1630–1635.

(2) Devor M. Neuropathic pain and injured nerve: peripheral mechanisms. *Br Med Bull* 1991;47: 619–630.

(3) Benarroch EE. Sodium channels and pain. *Neurology* 2007;68:233–236.

(4) Lai J, Porreca F, Hunter JC, Gold MS. Voltage-gated sodium channels and hyperalgesia. *Annu Rev Pharmacol Toxicol* 2004;44:371–397.

(5) Dib-Hajj SD, Cummins TR, Black JA, Waxman SG. Sodium channels in normal and pathological pain. *Annu Rev Neurosci* 2010;33:325–347.

(6) Cox JJ, Sheynin J, Shorer Z, et al. Congenital insensitivity to pain: novel SCN9A missense and in-frame deletion mutations. *Hum Mutat* 2010;31:E1670–E1686.

(7) Zochodne DW. Epineurial peptides: a role in neuropathic pain? *Can J Neurol Sci* 1993;20:69–72.

(8) Bove GM, Light AR. The nervi nervorum, missing link for neuropathic pain? *Pain Forum* 1997;6:181–190.

(9) Asbury AK, Fields HL. Pain due to peripheral nerve damage: an hypothesis. *Neurology* 1984;34:1587–1590.

(10) Levy D, Zochodne DW. Increased mRNA expression of the B1 and B2 bradykinin receptors and antinociceptive effects of their antagonists in an animal model of neuropathic pain. *Pain* 2000;86: 265–271.

(11) Donnelly-Roberts D, McGaraughty S, Shieh CC, Honore P, Jarvis MF. Painful purinergic receptors. *J Pharmacol Exp Ther* 2008;324:409–415.

(12) George EB, Glass JD, Griffin JW. Axotomy-induced axonal degeneration is mediated by calcium influx through ion-specific channels. *J Neurosci* 1995;15:6445–6452.

(13) Boivin A, Pineau I, Barrette B, et al. Toll-like receptor signaling is critical for Wallerian degeneration and functional recovery after peripheral nerve injury. *J Neurosci* 2007;27:12565–12576.

(14) Üçeyler N, Sommer C. Cytokine regulation in animal models of neuropathic pain and in human diseases. *Neurosci Lett* 2008;437:194–198.

(15) Üçeyler N, Tscharke A, Sommer C. Early cytokine expression in mouse sciatic nerve after chronic constriction nerve injury depends on calpain. *Brain Behav Immun* 2007;21:553–560.

(16) Kleinschnitz C, Brinkhoff J, Zelenka M, Sommer C, Stoll G. The extent of cytokine induction in peripheral nerve lesions depends on the mode of injury and NMDA receptor signaling. *J Neuroimmunol* 2004;149:77–83.

(17) Jung H, Toth PT, White FA, Miller RJ. Monocyte chemoattractant protein-1 functions as a neuromodulator in dorsal root ganglia neurons. *J Neurochem* 2008;104:254–263.

(18) White FA, Jung H, Miller RJ. Chemokines and the pathophysiology of neuropathic pain. *Proc Natl Acad Sci U S A* 2007;104:20151–20158.

(19) Levy D, Hoke A, Zochodne DW. Local expression of inducible nitric oxide synthase in an animal model of neuropathic pain. *Neurosci Lett* 1999;260: 207–209.

(20) Durrenberger PF, Facer P, Casula MA, et al. Prostanoid receptor EP1 and Cox-2 in injured human nerves and a rat model of nerve injury: a time-course study. *BMC Neurol* 2006;6:1.

(21) Ma W, Eisenach JC. Morphological and pharmacological evidence for the role of peripheral prostaglandins in the pathogenesis of neuropathic pain. *Eur J Neurosci* 2002;15:1037–1047.

(22) Ma W, Eisenach JC. Cyclooxygenase 2 in infiltrating inflammatory cells in injured nerve is

universally up-regulated following various types of peripheral nerve injury. *Neuroscience* 2003;121: 691–704.

(23) Vanegas H, Schaible HG. Prostaglandins and cyclooxygenases [correction of cycloxygenases] in the spinal cord. *Prog Neurobiol* 2001;64:327–363.

(24) Vergnolle N, Ferazzini M, D'Andrea MR, Buddenkotte J, Steinhoff M. Proteinase-activated receptors: novel signals for peripheral nerves. *Trends Neurosci* 2003;26:496–500.

(25) Vergnolle N, Bunnett NW, Sharkey KA, et al. Proteinase-activated receptor-2 and hyperalgesia: A novel pain pathway. *Nat Med* 2001;7:821–826.

(26) Asfaha S, Brussee V, Chapman K, Zochodne DW, Vergnolle N. Proteinase-activated receptor-1 agonists attenuate nociception in response to noxious stimuli. *Br J Pharmacol* 2002;135:1101–1106.

(27) Przewlocki R, Hassan AHS, Lason W, Epplen C, Herz A, Stein C. Gene expression and localization of opioid peptides in immune cells of inflamed tissue: functional role in antinociception. *Neuroscience* 1992;48:491–500.

(28) Stein C, Hassan AH, Przewlocki R, Gramsch C, Peter K, Herz A. Opioids from immunocytes interact with receptors on sensory nerves to inhibit nociception in inflammation. *Proc Natl Acad Sci USA* 1990;87: 5935–5939.

(29) Truong W, Cheng C, Xu QG, Li XQ, Zochodne DW. Mu opioid receptors and analgesia at the site of a peripheral nerve injury. *Ann Neurol* 2003;53:366–375.

(30) Chen Y, Sommer C. Activation of the nociceptin opioid system in rat sensory neurons produces antinociceptive effects in inflammatory pain: involvement of inflammatory mediators. *J Neurosci Res* 2007;85:1478–1488.

(31) Guindon J, Hohmann AG. Cannabinoid CB2 receptors: a therapeutic target for the treatment of inflammatory and neuropathic pain. *Br J Pharmacol* 2008;153:319–334.

(32) Guindon J, Hohmann AG. The endocannabinoid system and pain. *CNS Neurol Disord Drug Targets* 2009;8:403–421.

(33) Dray A. Neuropathic pain: emerging treatments. *Br J Anaesth* 2008;101:48–58.

(34) Vale ML, Marques JB, Moreira CA, et al. Antinociceptive effects of interleukin-4, -10, and -13 on the writhing response in mice and zymosan-induced knee joint incapacitation in rats. *J Pharmacol Exp Ther* 2003;304:102–108.

(35) Üçeyler N, Rogausch JP, Toyka KV, Sommer C. Differential expression of cytokines in painful and painless neuropathies. *Neurology* 2007;69:42–49.

(36) Wiesenfeld-Hallin Z, Xu XJ, Crawley JN, Hokfelt T. Galanin and spinal nociceptive mechanisms: recent results from transgenic and knock-out models. *Neuropeptides* 2005;39:207–210.

(37) Wilson-Gerwing TD, Dmyterko MV, Zochodne DW, Johnston JM, Verge VM. Neurotrophin-3 suppresses thermal hyperalgesia associated with neuropathic pain and attenuates transient receptor potential vanilloid receptor-1 expression in adult sensory neurons. *J Neurosci* 2005;25:758–767.

(38) Lewis T. The nocifensor system of nerves and its reactions. *Br Med J* 1937;27:431–494.

(39) Holzer P. Local effector functions of capsaicin-sensitive sensory nerve endings: involvement of tachykinins, calcitonin gene-related peptide and other neuropeptides. *Neuroscience* 1988;24:739–768.

(40) Lewis T, Harris KE, Grant RT. Observations relating to the influence of the cutaneous nerves on various reactions of the cutaneous vessels. *Heart* 1927;14:1–17.

(41) Cline MA, Ochoa J, Torebjork HE. Chronic hyperalgesia and skin warming caused by sensitized C nociceptors. *Brain* 1989;112:621–647.

(42) Lax H, Zochodne DW. Causalgic median mononeuropathies: segmental rubror and edema. *Muscle Nerve* 1995;18:245–247.

(43) Waller A. Experiments on the section of the glossopharyngeal and hypoglossal nerves of the frog and observations of the alterations produced thereby in the structure of their primitive fibers. *Philos Trans R Soc Lond B Biol Sci* 1850;140:423–429.

(44) Kennedy JM, Zochodne DW. The regenerative deficit of peripheral nerves in experimental diabetes: its extent, timing and possible mechanisms. *Brain* 2000;123:2118–2129.

(45) Verge VMK, Gratto KA, Karchewski LA, Richardson PM. Neurotrophins and nerve injury in the adult. *Philos Trans R Soc Lond B Biol Sci* 1996;351:423–430.

(46) Lawson SN. The peripheral sensory nervous system: dorsal root ganglion neurons. In: Dyck PJ, Thomas PK, eds. *Peripheral Neuropathy*. 4th edition. Philadelphia: Elsevier Saunders, 2005:163–202.

(47) Cummins TR, Sheets PL, Waxman SG. The roles of sodium channels in nociception: Implications for mechanisms of pain. *Pain* 2007;131:243–257.

(48) England JD, Gamboni F, Ferguson MA, Levinson SR. Sodium channels accumulate at the tips of injured axons. *Muscle Nerve* 1994;17:593–598.

(49) Faber CG, Hoeijmakers JG, Ahn HS, et al. Gain of function Nav1.7 mutations in idiopathic small fiber neuropathy. *Ann Neurol* 2012;71:26–39.

13

(50) Emery EC, Young GT, Berrocoso EM, Chen L, McNaughton PA. HCN2 ion channels play a central role in inflammatory and neuropathic pain. *Science* 2011;333:1462–1466.

(51) Chien LY, Cheng JK, Chu D, Cheng CF, Tsaur ML. Reduced expression of A-type potassium channels in primary sensory neurons induces mechanical hypersensitivity. *J Neurosci* 2007;27:9855–9865.

(52) Abdulla FA, Smith PA. Ectopic alpha2-adrenoceptors couple to N-type Ca2+ channels in axotomized rat sensory neurons. *J Neurosci* 1997;17:1633–1641.

(53) Abdulla FA, Moran TD, Balasubramanyan S, Smith PA. Effects and consequences of nerve injury on the electrical properties of sensory neurons. *Can J Physiol Pharmacol* 2003;81:663–682.

(54) Luo ZD, Chaplan SR, Higuera ES, et al. Upregulation of dorsal root ganglion (alpha)2(delta) calcium channel subunit and its correlation with allodynia in spinal nerve-injured rats. *J Neurosci* 2001;21:1868–1875.

(55) Newton RA, Bingham S, Case PC, Sanger GJ, Lawson SN. Dorsal root ganglion neurons show increased expression of the calcium channel alpha2delta-1 subunit following partial sciatic nerve injury. *Brain Res Mol Brain Res* 2001;95:1–8.

(56) Sills GJ. The mechanisms of action of gabapentin and pregabalin. *Curr Opin Pharmacol* 2006;6:108–113.

(57) Smith MT, Cabot PJ, Ross FB, Robertson AD, Lewis RJ. The novel N-type calcium channel blocker, AM336, produces potent dose-dependent antinociception after intrathecal dosing in rats and inhibits substance P release in rat spinal cord slices. *Pain* 2002;96:119–127.

(58) Snutch TP. Targeting chronic and neuropathic pain: the N-type calcium channel comes of age. *NeuroRx* 2005;2:662–670.

(59) Yaksh TL. Calcium channels as therapeutic targets in neuropathic pain. *J Pain* 2006;7:S13–S30.

(60) Altier C, Dale CS, Kisilevsky AE, et al. Differential role of N-type calcium channel splice isoforms in pain. *J Neurosci* 2007;27:6363–6373.

(61) Brittain JM, Duarte DB, Wilson SM, et al. Suppression of inflammatory and neuropathic pain by uncoupling CRMP-2 from the presynaptic Ca(2) channel complex. *Nat Med* 2011;17:822–829.

(62) Lieberman AR. The axon reaction: a review of the principal features of perikaryal responses to axon injury. *Int Rev Neurobiol* 1971;14:49–124.

(63) Zhang X, Bao L. The development and modulation of nociceptive circuitry. *Curr Opin Neurobiol* 2006;16:460–466.

(64) Ji RR, Zhang Q, Law PY, Low HH, Elde R, Hokfelt T. Expression of m, d, and k-opioid receptor-like immunoreactivities in rat dorsal root ganglia after carrageenan-induced inflammation. *J Neurosci* 1995;15:8156–8166.

(65) Li X-Q, Verge VMK, Johnston JM, Zochodne DW. CGRP peptide and regenerating sensory axons. *J Neuropathol Exp Neurol* 2004;63:1092–1103.

(66) Tsuzuki K, Kondo E, Fukuoka T, et al. Differential regulation of P2X(3) mRNA expression by peripheral nerve injury in intact and injured neurons in the rat sensory ganglia. *Pain* 2001;91:351–360.

(67) Frederick J, Buck ME, Matson DJ, Cortright DN. Increased TRPA1, TRPM8, and TRPV2 expression in dorsal root ganglia by nerve injury. *Biochem Biophys Res Commun* 2007;358:1058–1064.

(68) Xing H, Chen M, Ling J, Tan W, Gu JG. TRPM8 mechanism of cold allodynia after chronic nerve injury. *J Neurosci* 2007;27:13680–13690.

(69) Deval E, Gasull X, Noel J, et al. Acid-sensing ion channels (ASICs): pharmacology and implication in pain. *Pharmacol Ther* 2010;128:549–558.

(70) Bohlen CJ, Chesler AT, Sharif-Naeini R, et al. A heteromeric Texas coral snake toxin targets acid-sensing ion channels to produce pain. *Nature* 2011;479:410–414.

(71) Ramer MS, Murphy PG, Richardson PM, Bisby MA. Spinal nerve lesion-induced mechanoallodynia and adrenergic sprouting in sensory ganglia are attenuated in interleukin-6 knockout mice. *Pain* 1998;78:115–121.

(72) Murphy PG, Borthwick LA, Altares M, Gauldie J, Kaplan D, Richardson PM. Reciprocal actions of interleukin-6 and brain-derived neurotrophic factor on rat and mouse primary sensory neurons. *Eur J Neurosci* 2000;12:1891–1899.

(73) Murphy PG, Borthwick LS, Johnston RS, Kuchel G, Richardson PM. Nature of the retrograde signal from injured nerves that induces interleukin-6 mRNA in neurons. *J Neurosci* 1999;19:3791–3800.

(74) Murphy PG, Grondin J, Altares M, Richardson PM. Induction of interleukin-6 in axotomized sensory neurons. *J Neurosci* 1995;15:5130–5138.

(75) Ramer MS, Bisby MA. Adrenergic innervation of rat sensory ganglia following proximal or distal painful sciatic neuropathy: distinct mechanisms revealed by anti-NGF treatment. *Eur J Neurosci* 1999;11:837–846.

(76) McLachlan EM, Janig W, Devor M, Michaelis M. Peripheral nerve injury triggers noradrenergic sprouting within dorsal root ganglia. *Nature* 1993;363:543–546.

(77) Chung K, Yoon YW, Chung JM. Sprouting sympathetic fibers form synaptic varicosities in the dorsal root ganglion of the rat with neuropathic injury. *Brain Res* 1997;751:275–280.

(78) Suzuki R, Dickenson A. Spinal and supraspinal contributions to central sensitization in peripheral neuropathy. *Neurosignals* 2005;14:175–181.

(79) Zochodne DW, Murray M, Nag S, Riopelle RJ. A segmental chronic pain syndrome in rats associated with intrathecal infusion of NMDA: evidence for selective action in the dorsal horn. *Can J Neurol Sci* 1994;21:24–28.

(80) Nozaki C, Vergnano AM, Filliol D, et al. Zinc alleviates pain through high-affinity binding to the NMDA receptor NR2A subunit. *Nat Neurosci* 2011;14:1017–1022.

(81) Lim G, Wang S, Zhang Y, Tian Y, Mao J. Spinal leptin contributes to the pathogenesis of neuropathic pain in rodents. *J Clin Invest* 2009;119:295–304.

(82) Tian Y, Wang S, Ma Y, Lim G, Kim H, Mao J. Leptin enhances NMDA-induced spinal excitation in rats: A functional link between adipocytokine and neuropathic pain. *Pain* 2011;152:1263–1271.

(83) Coggeshall RE. Fos, nociception and the dorsal horn. *Prog Neurobiol* 2005;77:299–352.

(84) Tsuda M, Inoue K, Salter MW. Neuropathic pain and spinal microglia: a big problem from molecules in "small" glia. *Trends Neurosci* 2005;28:101–107.

(85) Coull JA, Beggs S, Boudreau D, et al. BDNF from microglia causes the shift in neuronal anion gradient underlying neuropathic pain. *Nature* 2005;438:1017–1021.

(86) Beggs S, Salter MW. Microglia-neuronal signalling in neuropathic pain hypersensitivity 2.0. *Curr Opin Neurobiol* 2010;20:474–480.

(87) Pernia-Andrade AJ, Kato A, Witschi R, et al. Spinal endocannabinoids and CB1 receptors mediate C-fiber-induced heterosynaptic pain sensitization. *Science* 2009;325:760–764.

(88) Dalal A, Tata M, Allegre G, Gekiere F, Bons N, Albe-Fessard D. Spontaneous activity of rat dorsal horn cells in spinal segments of sciatic projection following transection of sciatic nerve or of corresponding dorsal roots. *Neuroscience* 1999;94:217–228.

(89) Woolf CJ, Thompson SW. The induction and maintenance of central sensitization is dependent on N-methyl-D-aspartic acid receptor activation; implications for the treatment of post-injury pain hypersensitivity states. *Pain* 1991;44:293–299.

(90) Kohno T, Moore KA, Baba H, Woolf CJ. Peripheral nerve injury alters excitatory synaptic transmission in lamina II of the rat dorsal horn. *J Physiol* 2003;548:131–138.

(91) Sivilotti L, Woolf CJ. The contribution of GABAA and glycine receptors to central sensitization: disinhibition and touch-evoked allodynia in the spinal cord. *J Neurophysiol* 1994;72:169–179.

(92) Millan MJ. Descending control of pain. *Prog Neurobiol* 2002;66:355–474.

(93) Hudson AJ. Pain perception and response: central nervous system mechanisms. *Can J Neurol Sci* 2000;27:2–16.

(94) Zhuo M. Canadian Association of Neuroscience review: cellular and synaptic insights into physiological and pathological pain. EJLB-CIHR Michael Smith Chair in Neurosciences and Mental Health lecture. *Can J Neurol Sci* 2005;32:27–36.

Pain and carpal tunnel syndrome

Carpal tunnel syndrome is one of the most common acquired neuropathies and accounts for substantial disability with loss of time from work. Neuropathic pain is a prominent feature. In this vignette, we describe a patient with chronic symptoms of carpal tunnel syndrome in both hands and discuss the pain associated with this focal neuropathy.

Clinical case vignette

A 53-year-old right-handed female, working as a teacher, had experienced a 10-year history of symptoms in her hands. The symptoms initially involved the right hand but following a right carpal tunnel release, she began experiencing prominent left hand symptoms. These had been present for approximately 18 months and resembled her prior difficulties on the right. She described discomfort on the left at the severity level of 7/10 with tingling in the fingers, and burning, "pins and needles" at night, and electric-like shocks in the wrist and forearm. The electric shocks were provoked by grasping or picking up objects. Marking term papers of her pupils or using a computer exacerbated her discomfort. The symptoms might awaken her at night and in the morning. She noticed difficulty with her grip on the left. Her hand felt weak to lift, grasp, or carry bags but she had not noted paralysis of specific muscles. Her left hand felt cold and numb but she denied persistent loss of sensation. The patient had not tried using a wrist splint on the left.

There was no history of diabetes or thyroid disease. The patient reported chronic neck and lumbar discomfort. She could not generate sensory symptoms in her hands by moving or turning her neck. Her medications included celecoxib, cetirizine/pseudoephedrine, vitamins, and minerals. She had undergone bilateral mastectomies 1 year prior for carcinoma of the breast. Neither chemotherapy nor radiation had been administered. She had prior lower limb varicose vein surgery and right de Quervain's tenosynovitis.

The neurological examination of the upper limbs was normal. In particular, there was no Horner's sign and no weakness or sensory loss in either median nerve territory. The upper limb deep tendon reflexes were intact and symmetrical. There was no Tinel or Phalen sign.

Electrophysiological studies were completed in the upper limbs. In left median fibers, motor conduction was intact and the amplitude of the compound muscle action potential (CMAP) was normal. There was mild slowing of antidromic sensory conduction from the wrist to the index finger on the left with greater slowing from the wrist to the middle digit. Palmar conduction, with stimulation in the palm and recording over the wrist, was normal in the ulnar nerve distribution but there was significant slowing in the median territory. Left radial sensory and left ulnar motor and sensory conduction were normal. The left median and ulnar F wave latencies were within the normal range. On the right, median and ulnar motor and sensory conduction studies were essentially normal beyond borderline, likely residual slowing of right median palmar conduction. Overall the studies confirmed evidence of mild left-sided carpal tunnel syndrome involving sensory fibers.

The patient was scheduled for consideration of possible left carpal tunnel release by a plastic surgeon.

Pain description

The left hand pain involved the middle of the hand and radiated to the thumb and wrist. It also involved the fingers and forearm. The patient described the sensation as uncomfortable at 7/10; the tingling, burning, and electic shock sensations were exacerbated at night or with use of her hands.

Discussion

This patient's case description illustrates many key features of carpal tunnel syndrome (CTS). CTS is a focal neuropathy of the median nerve at the wrist. The carpal tunnel is a narrow passageway for the median nerve into the hand and is bounded dorsally (deep) by the concave surfaces of the carpal bones (hamate, capitate, trapezoid, and trapezium) and ventrally (under the skin) by the flexor retinaculum. The carpal ligament that roofs the tunnel is connected to the trapezium and scaphoid on the radial side and pisiform and hook of hamate on the ulnar side of the wrist. The median nerve shares the carpal tunnel with the long finger flexors of the hand, likely explaining why, as in our patient, wrist and finger movements can exacerbate the pain.

Risk factors for the development of CTS include pregnancy, repetitive hand work, diabetes mellitus, hypothyroidism, rheumatoid arthritis, local fractures and their associated deformities, amyloidosis, and anomalous muscles or blood vessels (1). In patients with a family history of bilateral CTS or other entrapment neuropathies, inherited sensitivity to pressure palsy (HNPP) should be considered.

In our patient, the condition was painful and interfered with her ability to work. The pain was centered over the wrist but radiated into her fingers and forearm. She experienced a sensation of hand weakness although no objective weakness could be demonstrated on her neurological examination. Many patients report that the symptoms involve the whole of the hand without localizing to specific fingers. Classically however, the sensory symptoms involve the median nerve territory, that is, the thumb, index, middle, and radial half of the ring finger. In the patient described here, clinical sensory examination was intact. Not all patients with CTS are noted to have a Tinel's or Phalen's sign and many patients with mild CTS do not have objective sensory deficits on examination. Many patients also report clumsiness and loss of hand dexterity. An important clinical finding in CTS is sparing of the territory of the palmar cutaneous branch that innervates the skin of the base of the thenar eminence and does not course through the carpal tunnel. Sensory loss in presumed CTS should, therefore, not include this territory. Bilateral CTS is common and should be routinely sought even in patients with unilateral symptoms. Because diabetes mellitus and hypothyroidism are important predisposing factors, these should be screened for in patients with CTS.

Decompressive surgery relieves symptoms of CTS more effectively than simple splinting but evidence for its benefit in CTS with either very mild symptoms or severe symptoms is uncertain (2). Approximately 75% of patients respond to carpal tunnel surgery (3). Surgery can identify other causes of median nerve compression at this level including anomalous muscles or vessels. Exposed median nerves that have been compressed may appear swollen, flattened, or inflamed (1). Corticosteroid injection relieves symptoms better than placebo (4) but it is argued that the benefit may only be short-term (3). Pre-operative electrophysiological studies improve the likelihood that the diagnosis is accurate and that the patient will benefit from decompression. Carpal tunnel release has been inadvertently carried out in patients with radiculopathy, motor neuron disease, syringomyelia, MS, and polyneuropathy (3). Thus, a careful diagnostic evaluation using electrophysiological studies is important.

Pain in carpal tunnel syndrome

The pain in CTS can be severe; some patients rank it as 10/10, it frequently reoccurs at night, and it can substantially limit their ability to work. The pain often appears to involve the whole hand as well as the wrist, forearm, and more proximal areas. Because axon damage may not necessarily complicate CTS, it is interesting to consider what generates the pain in this disorder. The pain does appear to be position- and use-dependent, suggesting a mechanosensitive local trigger. Mechanosensitivity is the basis for the Tinel's sign, the reproduction of characteristic clinical symptoms by mild tapping over the carpal tunnel. That many patients experience immediate pain relief and paresthesiae on decompression (1) is also remarkable, suggesting the presence of an ongoing peripheral nerve generator of the pain syndrome.

Atroshi et al. (5) examined 2466 people from the general population in Sweden who responded to a randomized survey. Approximately 14% reported pain, numbness or tingling in the median nerve distribution. Of these, approximately 5% of the original responders to the survey (approximately one third of those with symptoms) had electrophysiological evidence of median neuropathy and 2.7% had clinically and electrophysiologically confirmed CTS. In 125 control subjects without symptoms, electrophysiological studies identified asymptomatic CTS in 18%.

In some instances, painful mononeuropathy may be associated with segmental rubor (redness) and edema (swelling) strictly confined to the nerve

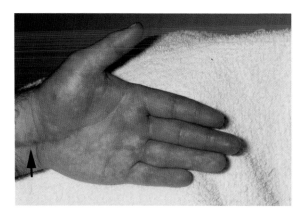

Figure 2.1. Rubor and swelling in a patient with CTS who had undergone decompressive surgery. Note the recently healed surgical scar (arrow). The patient had a complex pain syndrome (CRPS II) associated with his median mononeuropathy that was associated with severe pain, swelling, and localized color change. While the etiology for the localized changes is uncertain, recruitment of activity from peptidergic axons (expressing SP and CGRP) may contribute. This patient is described in reference (6).

territory in question. We described two patients with these tissue changes in association with "acute" median nerve injury at the level of the wrist in a previous report (6). The first patient had acute or chronic symptoms of CTS exacerbated by repairing her windows in her house. She described bilateral volar wrist pain, radiating proximally, rated as 10/10, followed by right median sensory loss, paresthesiae, and loss of hand power. She had a Tinel's sign, mild APB weakness without wasting, and loss of light touch and pinprick sensation in the median territory. There was striking hand and digital edema confined to the median territory. She had marked slowing and dispersion strictly across the carpal tunnel segment but no denervation to suggest axonal interruption. The symptoms largely improved with splinting and anti-inflammatory medication but she eventually did require carpal tunnel release over the next 2 years. The unusual facet of this patient was that the pain syndrome and edema changes resolved concurrently with improvement of demyelination (only) at the carpal tunnel. The second patient had sensory and motor abnormalities in the median nerve territory after a fall from a ladder onto his outstretched hand. Despite early carpal tunnel release, a pain syndrome ensued with cold sensation, color change, and swelling that was strictly confined to the median territory [Figure 2.1]. He improved spontaneously over time. This kind of syndrome might have been inappropriately termed "RSD" or reflex sympathetic dystrophy at one time but has more recently been classified as CRPS II (complex regional pain syndrome II); also known as "causalgia" in which a pain syndrome with soft tissue changes is associated with a local nerve injury. Ochoa and colleagues have described "angry" backfiring nociceptors that once activated by injury, cause antidromic release of peptides into the territory of the injury (7, 8). These peptides, including substance P (SP) and calcitonin gene-related peptide (CGRP), can be released locally by unmyelinated axon terminals and cause pain, edema from plasma extravasation, and vasodilatation.

"Failed" carpal tunnel release, with ongoing pain and disability, is an important complication. The most important cause is pre-surgical misdiagnosis, but incomplete release, adhesive neuritis, or intraoperative injury to the median nerve or the cutaneous sensory branch may also contribute to ongoing postoperative pain (9).

References

(1) Singh SK, Midha R. Carpal tunnel syndrome. In: Midha R, Zager EL, eds. *Surgery of Peripheral Nerves.* New York: Thieme, 2008:94–99.

(2) Verdugo RJ, Salinas RA, Castillo JL, Cea JG. Surgical versus non-surgical treatment for carpal tunnel syndrome. *Cochrane Database Syst Rev* 2008; CD001552.

(3) Bland JD. Treatment of carpal tunnel syndrome. *Muscle Nerve* 2007;36:167–171.

(4) Marshall S, Tardif G, Ashworth N. Local corticosteroid injection for carpal tunnel syndrome. *Cochrane Database Syst Rev* 2007;CD001554.

(5) Atroshi I, Gummesson C, Johnsson R, Ornstein E, Ranstam J, Rosen I. Prevalence of carpal tunnel syndrome in a general population. *JAMA* 1999;282: 153–158.

(6) Lax H, Zochodne DW. Causalgic median mononeuropathies: segmental rubror and edema. *Muscle Nerve* 1995;18:245–247.

(7) Ochoa JL. Essence, investigation, and management of "neuropathic" pains: hopes from acknowledgment of chaos. *Muscle Nerve* 1993;16:997–1008.

(8) Ochoa JL. The human sensory unit and pain: new concepts, syndromes, and tests. *Muscle Nerve* 1993; 16:1009–1016.

(9) Graham B. Recurrent or persistent symptoms following carpal tunnel release. In: Midha R, Zager EL, eds. *Surgery of Peripheral Nerves.* New York: Thieme, 2008:105–108.

Chapter 3

Pain and cervical radiculopathy

Cervical radiculopathy is one of the most common causes of neuropathic pain. Our clinical vignette describes a patient with cervical radiculopathy secondary to intervertebral disc protrusion associated with focal neuropathic pain.

Clinical case vignette

A 38-year-old right-handed man turned his neck to hear a sound while descending some stairs and developed an immediate pain in his neck and right shoulder. He rated its severity as 8/10, describing the pain as unlike anything he had experienced before. It had persisted for 3 weeks by the time of presentation to the Neurology service. The pain radiated into his right arm into the dorsal forearm, thumb, and index and middle fingers. These fingers also went numb, and he described a swollen, burning puffy sensation associated with them. He also described aching sensations, made worse with movement or straightening of his arm and further aggravated at night. Turning his head to the left increased the pain. A small dose of gabapentin (300 mg twice daily) was unhelpful. He denied symptoms in the left arm or in the legs, and there was no sphincter disturbance.

The patient had suffered a fall 8 years earlier with a diagnosis of left (opposite side from the current problems) brachial plexus injury but with no associated paralysis or sensory loss. He had otherwise been healthy and there was no prior history of neurological disease, neck surgery or injury. There was no family history of neurological disease.

On neurological examination, the patient had neck discomfort with reduced neck flexion and extension. There was no Horner's sign. The cranial nerves were intact. There was mild weakness of right elbow, wrist, and finger extension (Grade 4+/5 MRC). Other muscle groups had normal bulk, power, tone, and coordination. The right triceps reflex was absent but other deep tendon reflexes were present and symmetrical.

He had downgoing plantar reflexes. There was alteration to sensation to light touch and pinprick involving the right index, lateral middle, and thumb fingers partly into the forearm and a patchy change in the lateral arm above the elbow.

Overall, the clinical findings were highly suggestive of a right C7 radiculopathy with possible minor involvement of C6. Electrophysiological studies identified normal right and left median and ulnar motor and sensory conduction. Left and right median and ulnar F wave latencies were within the normal range. Needle electromyography of the right triceps, biceps, and extensor digitorum communis muscles were normal. Paraspinal muscle testing was deferred because of the patient's pain. MR imaging of the cervical intraspinal space [Figure 3.1] identified a right disc extrusion at C6–7 producing severe right neural foraminal stenosis. There was no significant spinal cord compression. The patient was referred for a spinal neurosurgical opinion regarding the possibility of a C6–7 discectomy.

Pain description

The patient described a swollen, burning, and puffy discomfort in the neck and right shoulder with aching into his forearm, thumb, and middle and index fingers. Movement, such as turning to the left or extension of the head, increased the pain. It was prominent at night. The pain was initially rated as 8/10 in severity but later diminished to 5–6/10. The regional localization of his pain, the association with neck discomfort and neck movement, and prominent involvement in a nerve root territory indicated radiculopathy with nerve root damage.

Discussion

Radiculopathies involving the C7 nerve root are the most common of the cervical radiculopathies (1). Radiculopathies can also develop in patients with multilevel cervical spondylosis that unfortunately are less

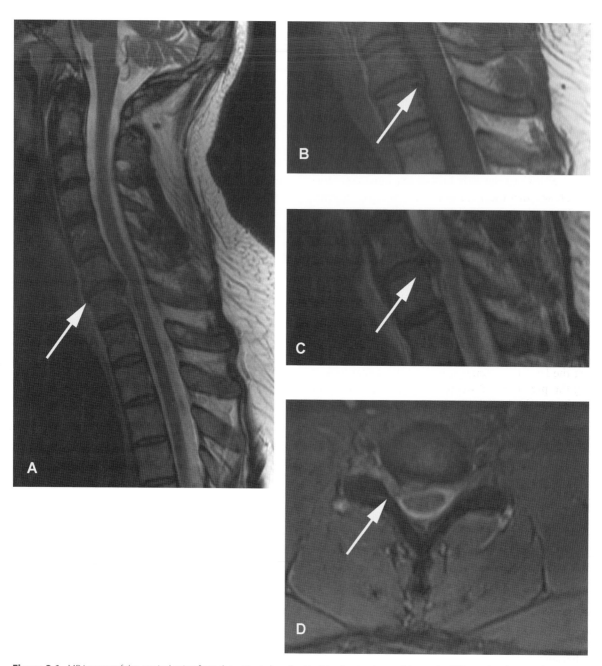

Figure 3.1. MR images of the cervical spine from the patient described in this chapter. Image A is a sagittal T2-weighted image showing a C67 disc protrusion impinging the cervical subarachnoid space. Images B and C show the disc protrusion at higher magnification on T1-(B) and T2-(C) weighted images. There was mild spinal cord indentation but no significant compression. Image D is a coronal view of the herniated disk showing loss of the foraminal subarachnoid space on the right side (arrow).

amenable to surgical therapy. One of the first and most comprehensive analyses of neurological symptoms from radiculopathy was provided by Yoss and colleagues who examined 100 patients at the Mayo Clinic in 1957 (2). C7 radiculopathy was associated with neck pain in 55% of the patients, scapular or interscapular pain in 37%, shoulder pain in 83%, lateral arm pain in 53%, and posterior arm pain in 34% of patients.

Our patient's descriptions of prominent shoulder and lateral/posterior arm pain mirrored these findings. In the Mayo series, 65% of patients had lost their triceps reflex and 65% had triceps weakness, findings identical to our patient. Finally, Yoss reported that only 24% of their overall series of patients had objective findings of sensory loss in the fingers, hand or arm associated with C7 radiculopathy. The same pattern of changes, including thumb involvement, was observed in our patient.

In all patients with radiculopathy, it is important to note whether there are symptoms or signs of spinal cord compression. This can occur from discs that herniate centrally into the spinal canal, from more chronic degenerative changes or from other causes. Spinal cord compression may be associated with sensory and motor symptoms in the lower limbs, difficulty with bowel or bladder sensation, and control and loss of balance. Lower (or upper) limb spasticity, weakness, hyperreflexia, upgoing plantar reflexes, and a sensory level may be identified on examination.

Electrophysiological studies are helpful in localizing the level of radiculopathy as well as characterizing the presence and degree of axonal degeneration in the involved territory. It may also exclude confounding conditions such as carpal tunnel syndrome or ulnar neuropathy at the elbow. Depending on the duration and degree of axonal involvement and the root involved, there may be loss of the amplitude of the compound muscle action potential (e.g., abductor pollicus brevis and abductor digiti minimi in C8 and T1 radiculopathies), preserved sensory nerve action potentials, and evidence of denervation in the involved muscles, including paraspinal muscles. These studies were normal in our patient, indicating that axonal damage had not occurred or was too early to detect. Given the 3-week duration of weakness, the absence of denervation in the weak triceps muscle may indicate that there was conduction block from demyelination in the proximal compressed C7 nerve root. This is because axonal damage and degeneration of the C7 nerve root within this time-frame should "normally" be associated with signs of denervation including fibrillations and positive sharp waves. Their absence, despite weakness, suggests demyelination of C7 without significant disruption of the nerve root axons. In other instances, frank denervation may be absent either because the interval between injury and sampling is too short (e.g., less that 10–14 days) or too long because reinnervation has already begun.

Progressive neurological dysfunction and intractable pain are the usual indications for possible surgical decompression (3), although high quality evidence of long-term benefits is limited, as addressed by a Cochrane review (4).

Pain in radiculopathy

Pain from cervical root damage occurs in 83/100,000 adults annually (5). As in our patient, it typically has a radiating or shooting quality often with an electric sensation. There are two main types of compression that often overlap. The nerve root and its associated dorsal root ganglia may be compressed by an osteophyte, a degenerative bony outgrowth in the foramina that causes narrowing. This problem, known as spondylosis, may account for up to 70% of cervical radiculopathies, especially in older patients. In younger people especially but overall in 20% of radiculopathies, intervertebral disc herniation may be responsible for nerve root and ganglia compression (3). Less common causes of cervical radiculopathy can occur and include tumors, cysts or infection.

Radicular pain may arise from one of several mechanisms: stretching of nerve sheaths or meninges as the root enters the spinal canal, ischemia, local root demyelination, local inflammation causing abnormal axonal excitability, or from changes in the intrinsic properties of nearby sensory neurons within dorsal root ganglia (DRG) due to compression.

There is evidence that DRG sensory neurons can develop abnormal excitability and generate spontaneous ectopic discharges associated with neuropathic pain (6). An experimental model of chronic compression of the DRG from foraminal stenosis was produced by insertion of stainless steel rods into the L4 and L5 intervertebral foramina of rats (7). At 5–10 days later, electrophysiological recordings from these neurons identified abnormal ectopic spontaneous activity in 10% of compressed neurons compared with only 1% of control uninjured neurons. Spontaneous activity was identified in large, medium, and small neurons and could be classified as type I activity, associated with subthreshold membrane potential oscillations and arising from the neuron soma, or less excitable type II activity without subthreshold oscillations and arising from the proximal axons within the ganglion. Abnormal spontaneous activity arising from compressed neurons was thought to produce "spurious" sensory information (e.g., paresthesiae).

21

Abnormal discharges could also be triggered by distal "physiological" stimuli (e.g., normal sensory stimulus), and these discharges could also block normal transmission. This may be analogous to descriptions in the clinical setting where patients with paresthesiae sometimes complain that normal sensitivity is altered by the presence of concurrent tingling sensations. In the model, ectopic discharges were tonic, bursting, or irregular. Type I activity was more commonly associated with bursting and type II with irregular discharges. All of these data indicate that at least two (soma, proximal axon) sites within the DRG can generate abnormal ectopic activity associated with neuropathic pain.

Inflammation in the area of the DRG may also promote abnormal spontaneous discharges of sensory neurons. For example, arachidonic acid is released from cell membranes by phospholipases present in the nucleus pulposus from a herniated disc. Arachidonic acid, in turn, is the precursor for prostaglandins (especially PGE2) synthesized by cyclo-oxygenase-2 (COX-2) that is expressed by inflammatory cells. Other algesic (pain generating molecules) that might generate inappropriate excitability of sensory neurons near a disc protrusion may include NGF, BDNF, interleukin 1β and 6, nitric oxide, TNFα, and others (see review by Van Zundert et al. (5)). In a model of noncompressive disc herniation in rats, altered gait accompanied mechanical allodynia, local inflammation, and autoreactive immune activation (8). In human herniated intervertebral discs, Shamji et al. noted greater interleukin-17 positivity, macrophage presence, and cellularity (9). In work using cultured human intervertebral disc cells obtained from patients scheduled for surgical disc therapy, exposure to IL-17, IFNγ, or TNFα showed an increase in their production of inflammatory mediators, nitric oxide (NOx), prostaglandin E2 (PGE2), interleukin-6 (IL-6), and intercellular adhesion molecule (ICAM-1); the findings identified an immunogenic phenotype (10). Thus, the intervertebral disc is described as immunogenic but both the DRG and the nerve root appear to require an additional mechanical insult to generate pain (11). In response to local inflammation, there may be secondary changes in sodium channel subunit expression that predispose neurons to increased ectopic firing, generating pain.

References

(1) Wilbourn AJ, Aminoff MJ. The electrophysiologic examination in patients with radiculopathies. *Muscle Nerve* 1988;11:1099–1114.

(2) Yoss RE, Corbin KB, MacCarty CS, Love JG. Significance of symptoms and signs in localization of involved root in cervical disk protrusion. *Neurology* 1957;7:673–683.

(3) Polston DW. Cervical radiculopathy. *Neurol Clin* 2007;25:373–385.

(4) Fouyas IP, Statham PF, Sandercock PA. Cochrane review on the role of surgery in cervical spondylotic radiculomyelopathy. *Spine (Phila Pa 1976)* 2002;27:736–747.

(5) Van ZJ, Harney D, Joosten EA, et al. The role of the dorsal root ganglion in cervical radicular pain: diagnosis, pathophysiology, and rationale for treatment. *Reg Anesth Pain Med* 2006;31:152–167.

(6) Wall PD, Devor M. Sensory afferent impulses originate from dorsal root ganglia as well as from the periphery in normal and nerve injured rats. *Pain* 1983;17:321–339.

(7) Ma C, LaMotte RH. Multiple sites for generation of ectopic spontaneous activity in neurons of the chronically compressed dorsal root ganglion. *J Neurosci* 2007;27:14059–14068.

(8) Shamji MF, Allen KD, So S, et al. Gait abnormalities and inflammatory cytokines in an autologous nucleus pulposus model of radiculopathy. *Spine (Phila Pa 1976)* 2009;34:648–654.

(9) Shamji MF, Setton LA, Jarvis W, et al. Proinflammatory cytokine expression profile in degenerated and herniated human intervertebral disc tissues. *Arthritis Rheum* 2010;62:1974–1982.

(10) Gabr MA, Jing L, Helbling AR, et al. Interleukin-17 synergizes with IFNgamma or TNFalpha to promote inflammatory mediator release and intercellular adhesion molecule-1 (ICAM-1) expression in human intervertebral disc cells. *J Orthop Res* 2011;29:1–7.

(11) Mulleman D, Mammou S, Griffoul I, Watier H, Goupille P. Pathophysiology of disk-related sciatica. I.–Evidence supporting a chemical component. *Joint Bone Spine* 2006;73:151–158.

Pain and diabetic lumbosacral plexopathy

Lumbosacral plexopathy, also known as diabetic amyotrophy, is a less common complication of diabetes than polyneuropathy and it can lead to devastating disability. This vignette describes a patient who had a relatively mild but recurrent version of this condition and exhibited spontaneous recovery. Some patients may be bedridden for several months with incomplete recovery.

Clinical case vignette

A 70-year-old man developed the sudden onset of severe sharp aching discomfort in his thighs. He had been diagnosed with type 2 diabetes mellitus 1 year earlier but had known glucose intolerance before that for 15 years. There was no history of retinopathy or nephropathy, and his glucose control had been good with fasting morning measurements in the 6–7 mmol/L range. The pain was predominantly limited to the right thigh with lesser symptoms on the left thigh. After the onset of pain, he experienced gradual loss of strength in his legs and eventually required the use of a cane. Neurological consultation was requested several months later. At 9 months following the onset of his difficulties, he reported that the pain had diminished to half of its former severity and his strength was slowly improving. Overall, he had also lost 23 lbs in weight. He had not experienced sensory loss but had noticed paresthesiae in both thighs. There were no upper limb symptoms. He also described erectile dysfunction, occasional postural lightheadedness, and constipation. There were no other sphincter difficulties.

His medications included nifedipine, gabapentin (600 mg divided in three doses), acetaminophen with codeine, and gliclazide. There was no prior history of hypertension, cardiac disease, or other systemic disorders. He had a previous hemorrhoidectomy, hernia repairs, varicocele, and left carpal tunnel release (15 years earlier). There was no relevant family history.

On neurological examination, he had mild intention tremor but the upper limbs were otherwise normal. He had wasting of the thighs, especially on the right, but normal bulk of extensor digitorum brevis muscles. There was weakness of hip flexors on the right (4+/5) and quadriceps (4/5), whereas other muscle groups in the right lower limb and all of the muscles in the left lower limb had normal power. Fasciculations were noted in the right thigh, and he had difficulty performing heel-shin testing on the right. All of the deep tendon reflexes, including ankle reflexes, were intact except an absent right quadriceps reflex. Sensation to light touch and pinprick was diminished in the right anterior thigh and medial leg below the knee in the saphenous nerve distribution. Sensation to vibration was diminished in the right toe. Sensory examination in other areas, including position testing, was normal. He had some difficulty walking tandem but could stand on his toes and heels. There was no Romberg sign. His blood pressure was 150/85 with a pulse of 88 supine and fell to 95/60, without a change in pulse, on standing.

An MRI of his lumbar spine and lumbosacral plexus identified mild central canal stenosis at L34 with ligamentum flavum and facet joint hypertrophy. There were no pelvic abnormalities. The right vastus lateralis had a mild increase in signal intensity on the inversion recovery sequences. Normal laboratory blood work included: hemogram, ESR, electrolytes, calcium, CK, serum protein electrophoresis, PSA, B12, and TSH. He had an elevated GGT level (502; normal, <50 U/L) but did admit to regular ethanol use. Barium enema, upper GI series, and abdominal ultrasound were normal.

The patient's use of gabapentin was associated with unacceptable dizziness, and he stopped the medication in favor of long-acting codeine and eventually long-acting morphine (MS contin 60 mg twice daily).

Electrophysiogical studies (10 months from onset) identified asymmetric CMAPs recorded over the vastus medialis (3.2 mV on the right; 7.2 mV on the left). Bilateral peroneal motor, bilateral tibial motor, right superficial peroneal sensory, and right sural sensory (amplitude 9.4 μV [normal, >6.0]; CV 41 m/s [normal, >39]) conduction studies were normal. Needle electromyography identified enlarged motor units in the right rectus femoris and tibialis anterior but no abnormal spontaneous activity (fibrillations or positive sharp waves). Right iliopsoas and L3/L4 paraspinal muscles were normal.

Seven months after his original presentation (16 months from onset), he developed bilateral ankle pain, a left foot drop, weakness of right foot plantar flexion, stocking and finger sensory loss, and had lost both knee reflexes and his right ankle reflex. He had maintained strict control of his glucose levels before these new symptoms. Repeat electrophysiology identified patchy but active denervation with fibrillations in the left tibialis anterior, right medial head of gastrocnemius, and enlarged motor units in the right tibialis anterior and left medial head of gastrocnemius without abnormal spontaneous activity. Rectus femoris was unchanged and there was no paraspinal denervation. Repeat imaging of the lumbar spine and lumbosacral plexus was unchanged. An ankle/foot orthosis was prescribed. Over the next few months, his new symptoms, including pain, improved, and he began to gain weight.

Five years after his original presentation, he had some persistent pain below his knees but his strength had largely recovered and bilateral ankle and knee reflexes had reappeared. He had distal foot sensory loss. He remained on a low dose of morphine (15 mg twice daily) and retained excellent control of his glucose levels.

Pain description

The patient described severe (10/10) sharp aching deep discomfort in his thigh that radiated into the tibial area and ankle. He also described the discomfort as burning. The initial symptoms were predominantly right sided.

Discussion

This patient developed an asymmetrical painful neuropathy largely involving the femoral nerve territory associated with mild type 2 diabetes mellitus. He also had sensory loss in the femoral and saphenous nerve territories. He had a prolonged biphasic neurological condition with a later exacerbation involving the con-

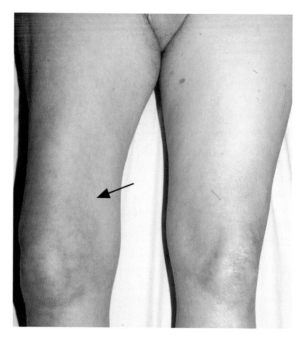

Figure 4.1. Proximal lower limb muscles of a patient with diabetic lumbosacral plexopathy. Note the wasting of the right (left side of image) thigh, particularly involving the vastus medialis.

tralateral peroneal nerve and ipsilateral tibial nerve. Only after the latter problem improved did he begin to regain his substantial weight loss. Imaging studies did identify mild lumbar canal stenosis but the findings were not sufficient to explain his prolonged progressive, then resolving course. He had no evidence of a connective tissue disease or vasculitis. When first seen, his pain and disability had slowly been improving.

The clinical features and course of this patient's condition are indicative of diabetic lumbosacral plexopathy (also called diabetic radiculoplexus neuropathy, asymmetric motor neuropathy, Bruns-Garland syndrome, or diabetic amyotrophy) (1). It is an uncommon but severe complication of diabetes mellitus and may develop despite optimal control of hyperglycemia, as observed in the present patient. Some instances may begin after initiation of insulin therapy. The condition is slowly progressive with prominent and intense deep aching thigh pain followed by atrophy and weakness of proximal lower limb muscles [Figure 4.1]. Severe lower limb weakness often confines patients to a wheelchair. Over the course of several months, the pain and then the weakness may resolve but symptoms may recur on the contralateral side or in other territories as with this patient. Weight loss, or cachexia, may be prominent and the course may be very prolonged, requiring hospitalization for pain control. Spontaneous recovery after many months is the typical outcome. Gabapentin was not helpful in our patient and, like many patients with this condition, opioid therapy was eventually required. Electrophysiological studies may identify denervation in the weak and wasted muscles including prominent paraspinal muscle fibrillations and positive sharp waves. There may also be widespread features of generalized diabetic polyneuropathy. The first electrophysiological studies for this patient were done 10 months into the course of his disease; at this time, fibrillations and positive waves had disappeared. He did have enlarged motor unit potentials indicative of prior denervation and reinnervation as well as loss of the amplitude of the CMAP recorded over the right vastus medialis. Acute patchy denervation was identified in other motor nerve territories during a later exacerbation.

The etiology of diabetic lumbosacral plexopathy is uncertain. Original descriptions, including a serial section pathological study through the lumbosacral plexus, emphasized infarction of nerve roots with occlusion of vasa nervorum (2). Several recent studies that have examined biopsies of the intermediolateral cutaneous nerves of the thigh described inflammatory vasculitis-like changes in nerve microvessels (3–6) [Figure 4.2]. Because clinical trial evidence is limited, optimal treatment plans are unclear; one series advocates the benefits of intravenous immunoglobulin while the experience of one of the authors (D.Z.) suggests the opposite (7, 8). A recent report has suggested that the use of corticosteroids facilitates rapid pain control but unfortunately, without an improvement in disability (9).

Pain in diabetic lumbosacral plexopathy

The pain experienced by patients with diabetic lumbosacral plexopathy is intense, prolonged, and difficult to treat. Opioid therapy may be required and hospitalization is frequent. The cognitive and gastrointestinal complications of chronic opioid therapy are problematic. The pain is typically reported to be deep within the thigh and precedes muscle weakness.

Several mechanisms may account for this unique pain syndrome. Its development early in the course of the neurological impairment, association with

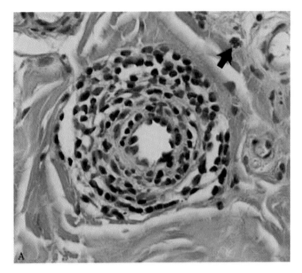

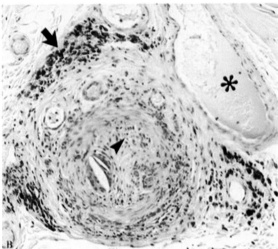

Figure 4.2. Transverse paraffin sections of sural nerves from patients with diabetic lumbosacral plexopathy as reported in Dyck et al. (6). In the top image (hematoxylin and eosin stain), an epineurial arteriole shows mononuclear cell infiltration within its wall. In the bottom image (Turnbull blue stain), another epineurial arteriole shows intimal thickening and proliferation (arrowhead), adventitial scarring, recanalization, and perivascular hemosiderin (arrow, blue). The asterix indicates fresh blood. The changes have suggested microvasculitis. Reproduced with permission from *Neurology* (6).

inflammation on nerve biopsy, cachexia, and response to corticosteroids all suggest a role for inflammatory cytokines. What repertoire of cytokines and chemokines may participate and why this inflammatory condition develops in the first place are unknown. Kawamura, Dyck, and colleagues (10) analyzed sural nerves from 19 patients with diabetic lumbosacral plexopathy and compared the findings with disease controls and biopsies from patients with nondiabetic lumbosacral plexopathy, an uncommon but similar condition. Nerve blood vessels had increases in ICAM-1 (intracellular adhesion molecule-1), whereas Schwann cells and macrophages had increased expression of TNFα. Both ICAM and TNFα are inflammatory mediators that may contribute to neuropathic pain. Infarction of the plexus alone might also lead to pain in this condition by generating ectopic discharges from injured nerves or activation of nervi nervorum, the unmyelinated axons that innervate the nerve trunk.

References

(1) Barohn RJ, Sahenk Z, Warmolts JR, Mendell JR. The Bruns-Garland syndrome (diabetic amyotrophy). Revisited 100 years later. *Arch Neurol* 1991;48: 1130–1135.

(2) Raff MC, Sangalang V, Asbury AK. Ischemic mononeuropathy multiplex associated with diabetes mellitus. *Arch Neurol* 1968;18:487–499.

(3) Dyck PJ, Windebank AJ. Diabetic and nondiabetic lumbosacral radiculoplexus neuropathies: new insights into pathophysiology and treatment. *Muscle Nerve* 2002;25:477–491.

(4) Said G, Goulon-Goeau C, Lacroix C, Moulonguet A. Nerve biopsy findings in different patterns of proximal diabetic neuropathy. *Ann Neurol* 1994;35:559–569.

(5) Said G, Elgrably F, Lacroix C, et al. Painful proximal diabetic neuropathy: inflammatory nerve lesions and spontaneous favorable outcome. *Ann Neurol* 1997;41: 762–770.

(6) Dyck PJ, Norell JE, Dyck PJ. Microvasculitis and ischemia in diabetic lumbosacral radiculoplexus neuropathy. *Neurology* 1999;53:2113–2121.

(7) Zochodne DW, Isaac D, Jones C. Failure of immunotherapy to prevent, arrest or reverse diabetic lumbosacral plexopathy. *Acta Neurol Scand* 2013; 107:299–301.

(8) Krendel DA, Costigan DA, Hopkins LC. Successful treatment of neuropathies in patients with diabetes mellitus. *Arch Neurol* 1995;52:1053–1061.

(9) Dyck JB, O'Brien PC, Bosch EP, et al. Results of a controlled trial of IV methylprednisolone in diabetic lumbosacral radiculoplexus neuropathy (DLRPN): a preliminary indication of efficacy. *J Peripher Nerv Syst* 2005;10 (Suppl 1):21.

(10) Kawamura N, Dyck PJ, Schmeichel AM, Engelstad JK, Low PA, Dyck PJ. Inflammatory mediators in diabetic and non-diabetic lumbosacral radiculoplexus neuropathy. *Acta Neuropathol* 2008;115:231–239.

5

Pain and meralgia paresthetica

Meralgia paresthetica is a common focal neuropathy of the lateral cutaneous nerve of the thigh in the upper lateral leg. Unfortunately, it is difficult to treat, particularly if it is associated with chronic neuropathic pain. This vignette describes a patient with painful bilateral meralgia paresthetica superimposed on chronic pain from osteoarthritis.

Clinical case vignette

A 49-year-old right-handed man experienced a 3-year history of burning pain in his legs, starting on the outside of the left thigh and associated with numbness. Two years after the onset, he noted similar burning pain involving the right lateral thigh with loss of sensation. He denied significant loss of sensation or pain in his feet.

His history was complicated by early onset and accelerated familial osteoarthritis that had interrupted his job as an oil field worker. He was unable to walk more than two blocks because of ankle and knee pain. There was no history of diabetes. He had undergone a cervical laminectomy at level $C_{5/6}$ 14 years earlier but no other lumbar surgery. A previous lumbar myelogram 6 years earlier identified multilevel degenerative changes and multilevel mild disc bulging without definite spinal stenosis. Although the patient had experienced several limb fractures in the past, he did not link any of these events to his ongoing pain problem.

Neurological examination identified changes to light touch and pinprick in the distributions of both lateral cutaneous nerves of the thigh; there was hypersensitivity to pinprick but loss of sensation to light touch. There was no analgesia or anesthesia. The remaining neurological examination, including quadriceps reflexes, was normal. There was no evidence of an inguinal lesion such as a lymph node or scar that might compress the lateral cutaneous nerves of the thigh. Notably, the patient did not have evidence of radiculopathy. He was overweight with central abdominal obesity. Other difficulties included depression and chronic abdominal pain.

Pain description

This patient described a pain syndrome rated as 10/10 in severity. He experienced joint pain unrelated to the neuropathy that accompanied burning pain in his legs along both thighs. His walking was very limited because of pain from both areas. Overall, his pain syndrome developed in the context of several other forms of somatic pain and disability including osteoarthritis and chronic abdominal discomfort.

Discussion

Meralgia paresthetica was diagnosed in this patient on the basis of clinical assessment without additional imaging or electrophysiological testing. The diagnosis was established by the distribution of the sensory alteration in the lateral side of the thigh with preservation of quadriceps motor power and the quadriceps reflexes. He did not have diabetes, a common predisposing condition to this neuropathy, but he did have abdominal obesity, thought to compress the nerve at the level of the inguinal ligament. Other local causes of nerve entrapment were not identified.

Meralgia paresthetica arises from local compression of the lateral femoral cutaneous nerve of the thigh. The nerve is a branch of the lumbar plexus arising from the L2 and L3 nerve roots and travels from the lateral side of the psoas major muscle over the iliacus muscle deep to its fascia. It passes into the thigh medial to the anterior superior iliac spine through a space beneath the lateral attachment of the inguinal ligament. It enters into the thigh anterior over the sartorius muscle with anterior and posterior branches that pierce the fascia lata to innervate the lateral thigh. There are variations in its course, however, described in other references (1, 2). These sources also list causes of the neuropathy that include compression

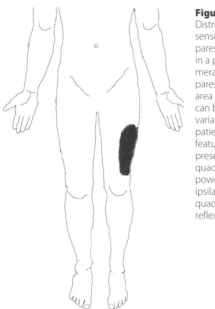

Figure 5.1.
Distribution of sensory loss, paresthiae, or pain in a patient with left meralgia paresthetica. The area of involvement can be highly variable among patients. Key features include the preservation of quadriceps motor power and an intact ipsilateral quadriceps (knee) reflex.

from obesity, pregnancy, ascites, local tumors, wearing heavy belts (such as toolbelts) or tight clothing, local hip pathology, inherited sensitivity to pressure palsy, diabetes mellitus, prolonged recumbency, injections, trauma, local surgery (hernia repair, appendectomy, iliac crest bone graft harvesting, others). Pelvic tumours and other lesions can target this nerve proximal to the inguinal ligament and injuries or injections can injure the nerve in the thigh. The nerve is not commonly targeted by vasculitis or other polyneuropathies beyond diabetes, in the author's experience. Occasionally, patients such as the one described in this vignette can have bilateral involvement if a predisposing cause, such as obesity, is present. The characteristic features are sensory loss, pain, paresthesiae, or a combination of these, involving the lateral thigh above the knee and below the hip [Figure 5.1]. The actual size of the area of involvement can be quite variable.

Thigh numbness and pain can also arise from L2–L4 radiculopathies; this patient had a known history of lumbar degenerative spondylosis. Radicular pain and associated radicular neurological deficits differ from those of meralgia paresthetica in that they often radiate from the back and are associated with loss of the quadriceps reflex (L3, L4 radiculopathies), muscle wasting, or weakness. Imaging studies of the lumbar intraspinal space or pelvis may be important to rule out other compressive lesions that involve the nerve roots or plexus. Often however, the preservation of

femoral territory motor power and a preserved quadriceps reflex clinically excludes most of these lesions. Relying exclusively on changes from imaging studies can be problematic because lumbar spondylosis is common in the general population. Moreover, an understanding of whether individual axons have been damaged as detected by imaging signal changes can only be guessed at. In our patient, there was concurrent lumbar spondylosis unrelated to his neurological problem. In instances where radiculopathy, plexopathy, or femoral neuropathy are suspected however, needle electromyography can be helpful; fibrillations and positive sharp waves in the involved territory may be identified. Paraspinal muscles may also show denervation in radiculopathies. There is no denervation of proximal lower limbs or paraspinal muscles in meralgia paresthetica. Although conduction studies of the lateral cutaneous nerve of the thigh are described and are possibly helpful in making a diagnosis, in the author's experience, these studies are less technically reliable than those of other nerve territories, particularly in obese subjects.

There is no high-quality clinical trial evidence to indicate that surgical decompression of the lateral femoral cutaneous nerve at the thigh is of greater benefit than conservative management. In some cases, the condition can resolve spontaneously over time. Despite these uncertainties (1), patients may choose to undergo decompression if weight loss, local anesthetic injections, or steroid injections are unhelpful and if pain is intractable.

Pain in meralgia paresthetica and other focal neuropathies

As in many focal neuropathies, the pain from meralgia paresthetica is typically more widespread than the actual sensory deficit. Pain may radiate proximally up the leg and below the knee. Because most instances of meralgia paresthetica arise from compression at and around the inguinal ligament, the symptoms are impacted by leg posture or walking. Pain is sometimes relieved by sitting to reduce the stretch or tension on the nerve. There may be painful paresthesiae that is roughly localized to the lateral thigh, with allodynia and accompanying lancinating or aching pains. A Tinel's sign over the nerve at the inguinal ligament may be present, also indicating mechanosensitivity.

The development of mechanosensitivity in focal areas of peripheral nerve damage is not fully understood. One important possibility is that impaired axoplasmic transport at sites of injury promotes the accumulation of mechanosensitive ion channels that generate ectopic activity. Dilley and Bove (3) generated mechanical sensitivity in unmyelinated axons by local blockade of axoplasmic transport without overt inflammation or axon damage. The authors postulated that specific accumulation of mechanosensitive channels proximal to the blockade was responsible for sensitivity. In additional work, they demonstrated that axoplasmic blockade proximal to a site of nerve inflammation prevented the development of mechanosensitivity.

Specific ion channels may be associated with the development of mechanosensitivity. Lewin and Moshourab (4) reviewed mechanisms of mechanosensation and describe roles for both C unmyelinated axons (C-mechanoheat, C-mechanocold, C-mechanosensitive, C-mechanoheatcold [polymodal] and C-silent, or mechanoinsensitive and thermal insensitive) and Aδ small myelinated axons (A-mechanosensitive with or without additional thermal sensitivity). Specific channels associated with mechanociceptor sensitivity may include the ASIC family (acid-sensitive ion channels; BNC1, BNaC1) comprising ASIC members 1–4. Mechanosensitivity in ASIC3 knockout mice is impaired (5). The involvement of TRP (transient receptor potential) channels in mechanosensitivity is also implicated. While the TRPV1, also known as VR1 or vanilloid, capsaicin-sensitive channel is the best known among this group, there are at least 33 TRP channel genes in mammals (6). TRPA1 channels, expressed in small-diameter nociceptive neurons, may be involved in the sensitivity to painful mechanical simuli. TRPV4 is yet another among this family of channels that may be similarly implicated.

Pain from focal neuropathies is well demonstrated in rodent models. Thermal hyperalgesia and mechanical allodynia in specific and standardized nerve injuries is extensively documented. The best known is the chronic constriction injury (CCI) model described by Bennett and Xie (7) that involves the placement of four loose ligatures around the sciatic nerve of the rat.

Over the course of the next few days, the underlying nerve segment develops swelling, ischemia from strangulation, and preferential damage to large myelinated axons. Rats (or mice) with CCI develop a shortened latency to withdrawal from a noninjurious thermal plantar paw stimulus and increased withdrawal and paw licking to stimulation with hairs of graded bending force (von Frey hairs). Despite extensive work using this model, analogous to many types of focal injuries in humans including meralgia paresthetica, the exact source of the pain generators is controversial. Axonal degeneration does not immediately ensue as in a crush or transection injury and spared small unmyelinated axons preserve sensation beyond the site of injury. Over time, regenerating axons may grow beyond and around the sutures and the pain syndrome disappears. Ectopic discharges can be recorded proximal to CCI, possibly due to contributions from both injured large myelinated axons and nearby uninjured C umyelinated axons. Nearby damaged axons may generate inflammation that promotes ectopic discharges either in C fibers en passant or from the intact ends of damaged large axons.

References

(1) Cook D, Midha R. Meralgia paresthetica. In: Midha R, Zager EL, eds. *Surgery of Peripheral Nerves*. New York: Thieme, 2008:167–170.

(2) Stewart JD. *Focal Peripheral Neuropathies*. 3rd edition. Philadelphia: Lippincott Williams and Wilkins, 2000.

(3) Dilley A, Bove GM. Disruption of axoplasmic transport induces mechanical sensitivity in intact rat C-fibre nociceptor axons. *J Physiol* 2008;586:593–604.

(4) Lewin GR, Moshourab R. Mechanosensation and pain. *J Neurobiol* 2004;61:30–44.

(5) Price MP, McIlwrath SL, Xie J, et al. The DRASIC cation channel contributes to the detection of cutaneous touch and acid stimuli in mice. *Neuron* 2001;32:1071–1083.

(6) Christensen AP, Corey DP. TRP channels in mechanosensation: direct or indirect activation? *Nat Rev Neurosci* 2007;8:510–521.

(7) Bennett GJ, Xie YK. A peripheral mononeuropathy in rat that produces disorders of pain sensation like those seen in man. *Pain* 1988;33:87–107.

6 Pain and Lyme radiculopathy (borrelia-associated radiculitis)

Several types of painful neurological problems may occur in Lyme disease, or borreliosis. This clinical vignette describes a patient with painful truncal radiculopathy that resulted from borrelia infection.

Clinical case vignette

A 66-year-old man developed pain of the left abdominal wall. He also complained of constipation. After consultation with his physician, a tentative diagnosis of diverticulitis was made and the patient was treated with the antibiotic ciprofloxacin. No improvement was observed after 2 weeks of treatment. Gastroscopy, colonoscopy, and colon barium x-ray studies were normal. His pain progressed and he developed numbness of the left abdomen. Tramadol, 200 mg per day in divided doses, was prescribed and provided moderate pain relief. MRI scans of the thoracic and lumbar spinal cord were normal. The patient was referred to the Neurology service because of his persisting numbness.

The patient's past history revealed a motorcycle accident with injury of the left brachial plexus and fractures of the left thigh and knee. He had no individual or family history of diabetes. Upon specific questioning, the patient remembered a tick bite approximately 4 months earlier but there was no history of rash that might suggest erythema migrans.

On general examination, there was no fever; the patient was obese but otherwise in good general health. On neurological examination, the patient had an abdominal wall paresis with bulging on the left side easily overlooked because of abdominal obesity [Figure 6.1a]. The cranial nerves were intact. There was mild weakness of shoulder abduction and elbow flexion and abduction (MRC grade 4/5) as residuum of the motorcycle accident. All other muscles had normal bulk, power, and tone. Coordination, stance, and gait were normal. Tendon reflexes were normal and symmetrical, plantar reflexes were downward. Sensa-

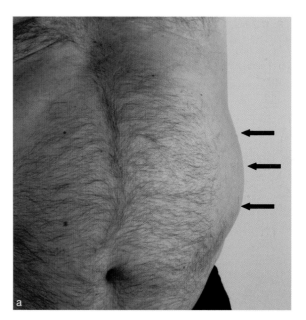

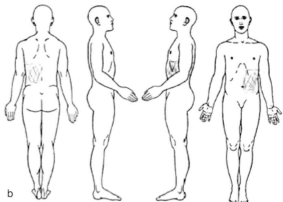

Figure 6.1. (a) Patient with left abdominal wall palsy due to borrelia infection. (b) Area of pain, patient drawing.

tion to light touch and pinprick was reduced in an area comprising the dermatomes T7 to T11 on the left [Figure 6.1b]. This was also the area where the pain sensation occurred. Light touch and pinprick

Tibial nerve SEP

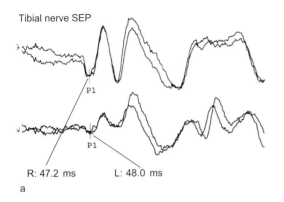

Tibial nerve MEP

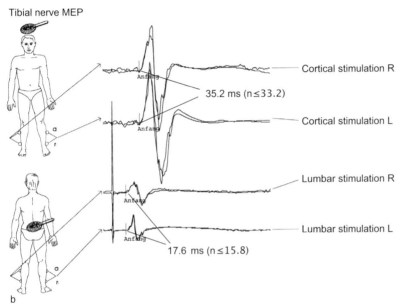

Figure 6.2. Original recordings of the patient's neurophysiological findings: (a) Tibial sensory evoked potentials (SEP) with prolonged latencies on the left. (b) Tibial motor evoked potentials (MEP) showed prolonged peripheral latencies bilaterally.

sensation were also reduced in an area over the left shoulder following the motorcycle accident.

Neurophysiological testing revealed prolonged latencies of tibial evoked sensory potentials on the left. Median nerve evoked sensory potentials were normal. Motor evoked potentials showed prolonged peripheral latencies bilaterally [Figure 6.2].

Routine laboratory tests were unremarkable. C-reactive protein was slightly elevated to 0.87 mg/dl (normal, 0–0.5). Glycosylated hemoglobin was normal as was an oral glucose tolerance test. Borrelia serology revealed a positive enzyme-linked immunosorbent assay (ELISA) for IgG and positive Western blots with several strong bands for IgG and IgM. Assuming radiculitis, lumbar puncture was performed, which revealed pleocytosis with 45 WBCs/µl, mostly lymphocytes. Cerebrospinal fluid glucose, albumin, and total protein were normal, and there were three identical oligoclonal bands in the CSF and serum. Borrelia ELISA was positive for IgG and Western blot showed two IgG bands. The CSF:Serum anti-*B. burgdorferi* antibody index was elevated with a value of 8.2 (normal, <1.4). A diagnosis of borrelia radiculitis (Lyme radiculitis) was made. The patient was treated with ceftriaxone 2 g/day for 3 weeks. A combination of sustained release tramadol 100 mg twice daily and pregabalin 150 mg twice daily provided pain relief. Complete recovery occurred over the next 3 months.

Pain description

The patient's overall pain intensity at initial presentation was rated as 6/10, despite treatment with tramadol. The patient described the pain as a constant burning with intermittent stabbing; it also had a deep aching component. Movement did not impact the severity of the pain. The pain was localized to the upper left abdomen. On the Neuropathic Pain Symptom Inventory (NPSI) (1), the patient characterized his pain as burning (6/10), squeezing (4/10), pressure-like (4/10), and stabbing (4/10). Overall pain intensity was reduced to 2–3/10 under combined treatment with tramadol and pregabalin.

Discussion

Painful paralysis of the abdominal wall muscles is a very uncommon clinical manifestation of Lyme neuroborreliosis. In a group of 90 patients suffering from early stage Lyme neuroborreliosis however, abdominal wall weakness was found in 11 cases (2). The lower thoracic segments (T7–12) are most often involved. Bilateral occurrence is not uncommon. Electromyography may show fibrillation potentials and positive sharp waves in paraspinal and abdominal wall muscles. Diagnostic errors are frequent, resembling the well-known descriptions of misdiagnosis that occurs in diabetic thoracoabdominal radiculopathy (2). Our patient was not diabetic. If the patient had been a diabetic, it is possible that lumbar puncture would not have been performed and the diagnosis missed or at least further delayed. Pain was the leading symptom, and the abdominal wall palsy was not evident to the first physician examining the patient, possibly due to the patient's obesity and to the relatively mild extent of the paresis. Furthermore, the patient complained of constipation. This constellation led to the consideration of diverticulitis that resulted in several unnecessary and partially invasive diagnostic measures, and delayed specific treatment. Elsewhere, cases mistaken for an acute abdominal crisis have been described (3). The differential diagnosis may also include post-herpetic neuralgia, and spinal disorders, as in fractured vertebrae due to malignancy; these were excluded by imaging in the present case.

Lyme neuroborreliosis develops in 15–20% of untreated individuals with borreliosis. The typical presentation is the combination of lymphocytic meningitis, cranial neuritis, and radiculoneuritis, as originally described (4). If meningitis is the leading syndrome, patients typically have headache and photosensitivity, are febrile, and CSF shows mild lymphocytic pleocytosis (mostly <100 WBCs/μl), mildly elevated protein, and normal or minimally decreased glucose. Cranial neuritis, often presenting as bilateral facial palsy, is another manifestation (3). Less common neurological manifestations include mononeuritis multiplex, distal symmetric peripheral neuropathy, brachial or lumbosacral plexopathies, myelitis with severe ataxia, and encephalomyelitis mimicking multiple sclerosis.

Given the typical history, clinical findings, and borrelia serology, the final diagnosis was unequivocal in this patient. The neurophysiological results also may have indicated a subclinical bilateral involvement. Parenteral ceftriaxone (2 g once daily) or cefotaxime (2 g every 8 h) for 14–28 days are established regimens for the treatment of neuroborreliosis. In European adults with Lyme neuroborreliosis, oral doxycycline 200 mg per day proved to be as effective as intravenous ceftriaxone (5).

It is still controversial whether infection with borrelia may lead to a syndrome encompassing chronic widespread pain and chronic fatigue (6, 7). Most experts argue that the assumption that chronic, subjective symptoms are caused by persistent infection with *B. burgdorferi* is not supported by adequate laboratory studies or controlled clinical trials, and that the use of prolonged, antibiotic treatments is not warranted (8).

Pain in radiculitis

Lyme radiculitis is typically painful, which does not help in differentiating it from compressive radiculopathy or diabetic radiculopathy. The pain is often burning, lancinating and strictly confined to the affected dermatomes. Paresthesias, allodynia, and hyperalgesia may occur in the involved region.

In terms of its pathophysiology, radiculitis pain is likely to consist of a combination of inflammatory and neuropathic pain. Unlike acute herpes zoster, another infection commonly leading to radiculitis, there are no experimental models of borrelia-associated radicular pain. Consequently, detailed knowledge of its pathophysiology is lacking. In the nonhuman primate model of Lyme borreliosis, inflammation localized to nerve roots, dorsal root ganglia, and leptomeninges was established (9). Infiltrating cells were mostly lymphocytes and B cells. Analogous to other types of nerve or root inflammation, spontaneous activity and sensitization of nociceptors can be inferred.

References

(1) Bouhassira D, Attal N, Fermanian J, et al. Development and validation of the Neuropathic Pain Symptom Inventory. *Pain* 2004;108:248–257.

(2) Pfadenhauer K, Schonsteiner T, Stohr M. [Thoraco-abdominal manifestation of stage II Lyme neuroborreliosis]. *Nervenarzt* 1998;69:296–299.

(3) Halperin JJ. Is neuroborreliosis a medical emergency? *Neurocrit Care* 2006;4:260–266.

(4) Garin C, Bujadoux A. Paralysie par les tiques. *J Med Lyon* 1922;71:765–767.

(5) Ljostad U, Skogvoll E, Eikeland R, et al. Oral doxycycline versus intravenous ceftriaxone for European Lyme neuroborreliosis: a multicentre, non-inferiority, double-blind, randomised trial. *Lancet Neurol* 2008;7:690–695.

(6) Cairns V, Godwin J. Post-Lyme borreliosis syndrome: a meta-analysis of reported symptoms. *Int J Epidemiol* 2005;34:1340–1345.

(7) Weissmann G. "Chronic Lyme" and other medically unexplained syndromes. *Faseb J* 2007;21:299–301.

(8) Feder HM Jr, Johnson BJ, O'Connell S, et al. A critical appraisal of "chronic Lyme disease". *N Engl J Med* 2007;357:1422–1430.

(9) Bai Y, Narayan K, Dail D, et al. Spinal cord involvement in the nonhuman primate model of Lyme disease. *Lab Invest* 2004;84:160–172.

Chapter

7

Neuralgic amyotrophy

Neuralgic amyotrophy, or brachial neuritis, is an intense inflammatory disorder involving the brachial plexus. Neuropathic pain at its outset can be very difficult to treat. In this vignette a patient with idiopathic neuralgic amyotrophy is presented, highlighting its typical course.

Clinical case vignette

A 25-year-old mechanic developed the abrupt onset of severe right shoulder pain. The pain was prominent at night and interfered with sleep. Ibuprofen offered little benefit. The pain disappeared a few days later, and the patient thought his problem had resolved. During the following weeks, he noted increasing weakness of his right arm prompting him to see a neurologist 2 months later. On examination, he had mild atrophy of all shoulder muscles and a winged scapula on the right [Figure 7.1]. There was weakness of all shoulder muscles on the right with an MRC score of 4-5. The right hand and finger extensors had mild weakness graded as 4+/5. Tendon jerks were brisk and symmetrical; pathological reflexes were absent. Sensation was completely normal for all modalities. Laboratory investigations, including cerebrospinal fluid analysis,

were normal. The EMG of the involved muscles did not show abnormal spontaneous activity and motor unit recruitment showed a mild neurogenic pattern. The patient was treated with oral prednisolone at 1 mg/kg for 10 days. The steroid was tapered over 4 weeks and then stopped. Pain did not recur. Regular physiotherapy was initiated. One year later, right arm strength had recovered, and the periscapular atrophy had largely recovered.

Pain description

The patient described his shoulder pain as very severe, unusual, and "like never before." An active sportsman, he had experienced previous injuries including an acromioclavicular joint injury on the left which resulted from a past skiing accident. He described his current pain as much more severe, equivalent to 8–9 out of 10. It was localized around the shoulder girdle, had started one night in the early morning hours and had reached its maximum within a few hours. The patient described the pain as deep, aching, and unlike anything he had previously experienced. Due to its severity, he could not sleep and spent most of the time sitting on the sofa. Ibuprofen and other NSAIDS did not alleviate the pain.

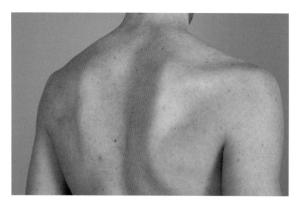
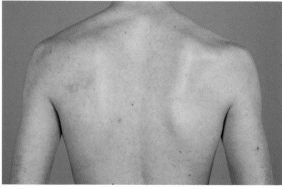

Figure 7.1 Winging of the right scapula in a patient with idiopathic variant of neuralgic amyotrophy.

Discussion

Neuralgic amyotrophy was described in 1948 by Parsonage and Turner, who identified 136 cases between 1941 and 1945. Synonyms for this disorder include Parsonage-Turner syndrome, plexus neuritis, sporadic brachial plexus neuropathy, and neuralgic amyotrophy (NA). Both idiopathic (INA) and hereditary variant (HNA) forms occur. INA has an incidence of 1–4/100,000, comparable to Guillain-Barré syndrome. HNA is rare and has been described in approximately 200 families worldwide. Men are more afflicted than women, in a ratio of 3:2. INA occurs most often in the second to fourth decade of life, HNA in the second decade. Onset at any age is possible, particularly in the case of INA. The clinical picture typically consists of acute and very severe shoulder–arm pain that remits over days or weeks followed by multifocal atrophic pareses in the same region. The interval between the onset of pain and the development of weakness varies between under 24 h to over 2 weeks. Rare forms without pain (1) have also been reported.

The weakness of INA may involve all parts of the brachial plexus. In 70% of cases, the upper plexus is involved. Sensory deficits may be present and may not correspond to the anatomical distribution of the motor deficits. This patchy pattern is a helpful diagnostic sign. The contralateral arm has mild involvement in a third of all patients. Therefore, a full neurological examination with testing of muscle strength in apparently unaffected muscles is necessary. The typical motor pattern is that of an upper brachial plexus lesion. The periscapular and perihumeral muscles are involved in 70% of men. The long thoracic nerve is involved in two thirds of patients, often leading to winging of the scapula (Figure 1). The lower plexus is involved in approximately 25% of women and 10% of men.

While the brachial plexus is predominantly affected in INA, 60% of HNA patients have involvement of the lumbosacral plexus, involved in only 17% of INA patients. Rarely, the phrenic nerve, the facial nerve, and abdominal nerves may be involved. The medial and lateral antebrachial cutaneous nerves, which innervate the volar forearm, may also be impacted because they emerge directly from the brachial plexus. This causes pain and a sensory deficit of the volar forearm. SNAP amplitudes may be reduced. Hyperintense areas of the brachial plexus in T2-weighted MRI scans have been reported. Because this finding is only present in approximately 10% of cases however, it has a very low sensitivity for the diagnosis of INA. In contrast, MRI of the shoulder musculature may delineate the pattern of wasted involved muscles. Imaging may also help determine prognosis (2).

Laboratory testing is unhelpful. The presence of anti-ganglioside antibodies has been described. CSF rarely reveals increased protein levels or oligoclonal bands. EMG shows signs of denervation and reinnervation in the involved muscles. In nerve conduction studies, CMAP amplitudes are only reduced when muscles are significantly weak although asymmetrically reduced CMAP responses may accompany fibrillation potentials and positive sharp waves. The differential diagnosis of brachial plexus lesion includes trauma, radiation, Pancoast tumor, thoracic outlet syndrome, and infectious causes such as neuroborreliosis and HIV.

Pain in neuralgic amyotrophy

Apart from specific tests that eliminate alternative differential diagnoses in patients with INA, specific pain characteristics are very helpful in distinguishing it from other manifestations of shoulder disease (1). If the pain is acute, very severe, and unlike anything the patient has previously experienced, a diagnosis of INA is very likely. If not, NA is possible but alternative pathologies should be considered. With limited passive arm external rotation or abduction, shoulder joint pathology such as bursitis or tendinitis is more likely. If the pain is in the same root distribution as the symptoms (paresis, sensory disturbances), cervical radiculopathy should be considered. In 90% of patients, the disorder starts with an unusual, very severe pain in the shoulder–arm area that reaches maximum severity within a few hours. The duration of severe or moderate pain can range from less than 24 h to persisting for several months. Standard analgesics have no effect. Patients describe the pain as unusually severe, radiating from the shoulder to the neck and to the arm. In 60%, the onset occurs when the patient is at rest or sleeping, and remains severe at night interfering with sleep. When asked to quantify the pain, patients usually mark scores between 7 and 10 out of 10. Up to 80% of patients report some pain, although milder, at the onset of the weakness. On examination, the pain is increased by elevating and abducting the arm; this has been termed, "the Lasègue sign of the arm." The pain usually remits within weeks to months. In the acute phase, the inflammatory aspect of the pain predominates. Within days to weeks, this leads to a second phase which is considered mostly neuropathic and is characterized by spontaneous or movement-induced shooting pain and tingling sensations in the anatomical distribution of the plexus. Once the acute pain has subsided, a different, musculoskeletal type of pain, caused by muscular instability at the shoulder joint may develop. Patients with instability of the scapula due to paresis of the serratus anterior, rhomboid, or trapezius muscle and with instability of the rotator cuff have a higher risk for developing this musculoskeletal pain.

INA is regarded as an auto-immune disorder (1). As observed in Guillain-Barré syndrome, specific events appear to trigger an immune response in approximately 50% of cases. These include infections, surgery, pregnancy, mental and physical stress, immunizations, and immunodulating therapies. Mechanical factors may also be a risk factor. Because approximately 50% of patients do not report a preceding event, other factors must also be considered. In HNA, this requires review of the genetic background. In approximately 55% of families, the gene for HNA has been localized to the SEPT9 gene on human chromosome 17q25.3 (3, 4). Septins are highly conserved filamentous proteins. The SEPT9 mutation may regulate interactions of septin-9 with other septins or other cellular proteins (5), but the mechanism by which it leads to HNA is unknown.

In the acute phase, a combination of a long-acting NSAID and an opiate, such as diclofenac 100 mg bid and 10–30 mg of a slow release morphine, is recommended. An NSAID alone is often not sufficient. In the second phase when the neuropathic component is predominant, drugs prescribed for neuropathic pain may be helpful. They include pregabalin, gabapentin, amitriptyline, or carbamazepine. Case reports have linked the use of oral prednisolone to faster pain relief and recovery in strength (6). Other immune treatments appear to have no effect (7).

During the third, musculoskeletal phase of pain which can vary in duration, pharmacological treatment has little effect. A combination of physical therapy and adaptation to activities of daily life is recommended (1). It is important that involved muscles are not overused and further damaged. Secondary joint pathology, such as irritation of the rotator cuff, bursitis or cuff tendon rupture, requires orthopedic intervention.

References

(1) van Alfen N. The neuralgic amyotrophy consultation. *J Neurol* 2007;254:695–704.

(2) Scalf RE, Wenger DE, Frick MA, Mandrekar JN, Adkins MC. MRI findings of 26 patients with Parsonage-Turner syndrome. *AJR Am J Roentgenol* 2007;189:W39–W44.

(3) Pellegrino JE, Rebbeck TR, Brown MJ, Bird TD, Chance PF. Mapping of hereditary neuralgic amyotrophy (familial brachial plexus neuropathy) to distal chromosome 17q. *Neurology* 1996;46: 1128–1132.

(4) Hannibal MC, Ruzzo EK, Miller LR, et al. SEPT9 gene sequencing analysis reveals recurrent mutations in hereditary neuralgic amyotrophy. *Neurology* 2009; 72:1755–1759.

(5) Nagata K, Asano T, Nozawa Y, Inagaki M. Biochemical and cell biological analyses of a mammalian septin complex, Sept7/9b/11. *J Biol Chem* 2004;279:55895–55904.

(6) van Eijk JJ, van Alfen N, Berrevoets M, van der Wilt GJ, Pillen S, van Engelen BG. Evaluation of prednisolone treatment in the acute phase of neuralgic amyotrophy: an observational study. *J Neurol Neurosurg Psychiatry* 2009;80:1120–1124.

(7) van Alfen N, van Engelen BG, Hughes RA. Treatment for idiopathic and hereditary neuralgic amyotrophy (brachial neuritis). *Cochrane Database Syst Rev* 2009:CD006976.

Painful radiculopathy associated with herpes zoster infection

Herpes zoster is associated with one of the most intense neuropathic pain syndromes. The virus is associated with pain in the territory of one or more adjacent nerve roots, most commonly on the trunk but occasionally involving cervical and lumbar root distributions. Pain and a vesicular rash may be associated with motor weakness and denervation in the territory involved. Zoster-related neuropathic pain has figured prominently in clinical trials but often is refractory to treatment.

Clinical case vignette

A 72-year-old right-handed female developed neck and shoulder discomfort after attending a wedding. Chiropractic "cupping" failed to alleviate the pain, and she developed a vesicular rash involving the lateral side of her right neck, right posterior shoulder, posterior arm, and volar forearm. She was treated with valcyclovir. The rash persisted for approximately 6 weeks before healing. The skin lesions were associated with both superficial and deep pain rated as 8–9/10 in severity.

As the vesicles presented, the patient developed weakness lifting her arm up or bending at the elbow. She had difficulty combing her hair, feeding herself, and raising her arm. She noted tingling from her right shoulder radiating down her arm and into her thumb with sensory loss in a similar distribution.

There had been no prior episodes of herpes zoster. She had been in good health and there was no history of diabetes mellitus, malignancy, or immunosuppression. Medications included synthroid, gabapentin, vitamins, acetaminophen with codeine, and losartan.

On examination at 3 months following her initial symptoms, she had healed scars characteristic of herpes zoster involving the right lateral neck, anteromedial arm, and volar forearm including the antebrachial area. She had weakness of the right deltoid (2/5), right biceps (3–/5) with an intact brachioradialis, triceps, and other right upper limb muscles. The left arm and lower limbs were intact. The right biceps and brachioradialis reflexes were absent. On sensory examination, there was loss to light touch and pinprick over the anterior forearm, medial arm, and lateral shoulder. There were no other neurological findings.

Electrophysiological studies identified a reduction in the amplitude of the compound muscle action potential recorded over the right deltoid muscle on stimulation of the axillary nerve. Needle electromyography identified abnormal spontaneous activity with fibrillations and positive sharp waves in the right deltoid, biceps, and right C6 paraspinal muscles. There were reduced numbers of motor unit potentials recorded from the right deltoid muscle and to a lesser extent in the right biceps. Overall, the findings were indicative of a right C5–6 radiculopathy secondary to herpes zoster radiculitis.

MR imaging identified a signal abnormality involving the cervical spinal cord from C2–3 to C6–7 involving the central gray matter including the anterior and posterior horns with sparing of peripheral white matter [Figure 8.1A]. The changes primarily involved the right hemicord where mild enhancement was observed. There was no cord edema. Osteophytes and foraminal stenosis were also identified at several levels and on both sides of the cervical spine (C34, C45, C56).

The weakness persisted over the next 6 weeks with the onset of slow and gradual improvement after that. Burning superficial discomfort persisted for 6 months after the onset of the rash. By 9 months after the rash, she could comb her hair, and by 10 months, she reported only 75% of her baseline strength. Recovery was complicated by a pre-existing diagnosis of painless rotator cuff impingement in the same arm.

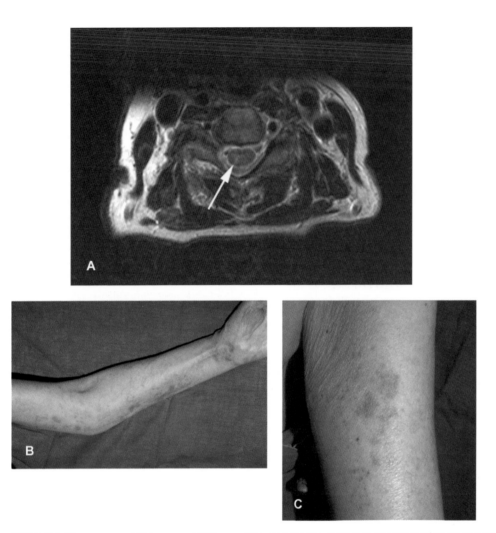

Figure 8.1. The upper panel (A) is a coronal MR image of the cervical spine at approximately the level C4 (T2 weighted) showing a signal change involving the right side of the spinal cord extending from the dorsal horn into the anterior gray matter (arrow). The photographs in (B) and (C) illustrate examples of healed scars from herpes zoster in a separate patient that had involvement of the C8 and T1 nerve root distributions with associated motor weakness in the hand and forearm.

Pain description

The patient had no previous history of arm pain. She reported superficial burning discomfort that she rated as 9/10 in severity and that was distributed over the same area as the rash. The pain outlasted the rash however, persisting for 6 months in total. It was exacerbated by contact with clothing or the bed covers and by movement. The pain was present day and night without remit and interfered with her ability to sleep; she was unable to lie on her side with her head propped up. A second type of pain was described as deep and aching, of similar severity radiating from her neck into her shoulder, upper arm, and forearm. By 10 months after the onset of the rash, this pain was persistent and was exacerbated by use and movement. At this time, it was rated as 2–3/10 in severity.

Analgesic medications had been helpful, but their actions were incomplete. An initial trial of gabapentin up to 2400 mg daily was associated with cognitive side effects. Pregabalin was more effective but induced lower limb edema. Acetaminophen/oxycodone was helpful. By 10 months, she was still using codeine contin and acetaminophen with codeine.

Discussion

The patient presented with features of herpes zoster radiculitis of the C5–C6 distribution with the initial onset of severe pain followed by the outbreak of a characteristic rash. The rash was described as clusters of papules that developed into vesicles on an erythematous base. Although some instances of zoster radiculitis occur in the absence of rash ("zoster sine herpete"), the characteristic rash, sensory symptoms, and pain follow a segmental distribution involving one or more adjacent root territories. Pain from early truncal herpes zoster may incorrectly suggest an abdominal or thoracic emergency. In this patient, the diagnostic features involved the C5 and C6 skin sensory territories over the shoulder and upper arm with some sensory symptoms radiating into the thumb. The patient's description of neuropathic pain with zoster was characteristic and included superficial burning with allodynia, but also deep discomfort. In addition to the exquisite pain syndrome associated with zoster, segmental involvement of motor neurons can also develop with denervation, as identified in this patient, in the territory of sensory symptoms and rash. The patient had relatively mild motor involvement but denervation in other territories can be severe rendering foot drop, hand paralysis, and other deficits depending on the level of involvement. Needle electromyography is helpful in mapping out the distribution of the denervation. In this case, paraspinal muscle involvement indicated a proximal level of involvement at the root or segmental gray matter. Imaging studies confirmed segmental signal change in the spinal cord on the side of involvement. Given the persistent nature of the discomfort over many months, she later fulfilled the diagnosis of post-herpetic neuralgia. Our patient did not have diabetes mellitus or immunosuppression, but her older age was a risk factor.

Herpes zoster arises from human infection with a neurotropic alpha-herpesvirus. It is a common disorder with an incidence at 5–6.5 per 1000 but its incidence increases with age and may occur in up to 11 per 1000 persons by the age of 70 (1). The pain associated with herpes zoster arises from an acute inflammatory reaction that involves one or more adjacent segmental sensory dorsal root ganglia (or sensory cranial nerves) with extension into nerve roots. Segmental mild leptomeningeal inflammation is common and acutely infected ganglia have direct evidence of herpes zoster virus invasion. Inflammation can also extend into the posterior horn of the spinal cord, and less commonly into the anterior horn rendering "poliomyelitis" (inflammation of gray matter). In acute zoster, pain usually lasts for 1–6 weeks with resolution of the rash (small cutaneous scars may remain) (2). After the lesions have healed, scars may be evident in the nerve root territory involved [Figure 8.1B,C].

Painful herpes zoster radiculitis or cranial neuritis is only one of several complications of zoster infection of the nervous system which includes vasculopathy, myelopathy, and retinal necrosis. Vasculopathy may be associated with focal ischemic neurological deficits and cerebral hemorrhage. Facial nerve zoster is associated with facial paralysis (Ramsay Hunt syndrome) and trigeminal zoster is a medical emergency (herpes zoster ophthalmicus). Zoster sine herpete exhibits segmental or radicular pain in the absence of a rash. While the existence of this syndrome has been in some doubt historically, several recent cases have confirmed infection in the clinical syndrome without rash (2, 3). Acute zoster is treated with antiviral agents and analgesics. Childhood varicella vaccination may lead to a reduction in the prevalence of herpes zoster and in 2006, a new zoster vaccine was approved by the FDA for healthy adults over 60 years of age who are seropositive for the virus (2).

Pain associated with herpes zoster infection

Post-herpetic neuralgia occurs in 40% of zoster patients over the age of 60 (4) and is defined as pain that persists for at least 3 months after the disappearance of the rash. The exact mechanisms through which zoster generates pain is uncertain, but a role for local ganglion virus reactivation and ganglionitis has been considered. For example, up to 7% of DRG neurons may contain latent virus (2). Associated mechanisms likely involve altered properties of surviving neuron subpopulations that may predispose a pain phenotype. These include a shift in the excitability characteristics of residual neurons, long-term plastic changes of neuronal sodium or calcium channels, persistent DRG infiltration of inflammatory cells with inflammatory cytokines, TNFα or free-radicals, or finally, alterations in the behavior of perineuronal glial cells. Because the inflammation of herpes zoster often involves leptomeninges and the dorsal horn of the spinal cord, altered dorsal horn circuitry, as occurs after simple axotomy injuries or peripheral inflammatory lesions, may also play an important role. The burning phenotype combined with striking allodynia argues for mechanisms that involve smaller caliber nociceptive neurons, but also remodeling of normally non-nociceptive pathways that usually involve light touch to mediate allodynia.

References

(1) Donahue JG, Choo PW, Manson JE, Platt R. The incidence of herpes zoster. *Arch Intern Med* 1995;155:1605–1609.

(2) Mueller NH, Gilden DH, Cohrs RJ, Mahalingam R, Nagel MA. Varicella zoster virus infection: clinical features, molecular pathogenesis of disease, and latency. *Neurol Clin* 2008;26:675–697, viii.

(3) Blumenthal DT, Shacham-Shmueli E, Bokstein F, et al. Zoster sine herpete: virologic verification by detection of anti-VZV IgG antibody in CSF. *Neurology* 2011;76:484–485.

(4) Rogers RS, III, Tindall JP. Herpes zoster in the elderly. *Postgrad Med* 1971;50:153–157.

Pain and chronic inflammatory demyelinating polyneuropathy

Chronic inflammatory demyelinating polyneuropathy (CIDP) is a progressive or relapsing disorder of peripheral nerves associated with prominent motor involvement. This vignette describes a patient with CIDP who experienced severe neuropathic pain. The diagnosis at outset was challenging and his condition (and pain) progressed because he declined ongoing therapy.

Clinical case vignette

A 51-year-old right-handed construction worker had a 6-year history of burning tingling sensations that began in his feet from the ankle down and then progressed to involve the posterior calf. He experienced cramping in his feet or legs and developed loss of sensation with paresthesiae of his legs. During the year before his assessment, he had noted a decline in balance, difficulty lifting his feet, numbness in his fingertips, and burning in his forearms.

The patient had undergone two prior lumbar laminectomies, the first 25 years earlier and the second, 1 year later. The second procedure did not improve his symptoms. He had been treated out of the country with prednisone and cyclophosphamide for a possible inflammatory neuropathy, although a firm diagnosis had not been established. He had remote removal of an abdominal paraganglioma. He was taking diazepam but no other medications. There was no history of diabetes, hypertension, or significant systemic disease, and there was no family history of polyneuropathy. A brother was later diagnosed with ALS.

On neurological examination, he had loss of muscle bulk below his knees, effort-limited voluntary muscle recruitment but otherwise normal muscle power throughout. He was areflexic. On sensory examination, there was loss of sensation to light touch, pinprick, cold sensation, and vibration perception in his feet to the mid-tibia and in his fingers. His toes were anesthetic and analgesic. He could stand on his toes and heels but had an unusual lurching gait, improved with using a cane.

After his initial visit, the patient was followed intermittently for 14 years in clinic. His ongoing neurological care was significantly complicated by long absences out of the country, depression, and very limited compliance with treatment regimens. His overall course was that of gradual deterioration and increasing neuropathic pain, despite some periods of improvement while on immunosuppressive medication. Four years after initial evaluation, he required a cane to ambulate. His first set of electrophysiological studies in our clinic identified patchy slowing of motor conduction velocity in his ulnar and peroneal nerves and diffuse loss of sensory nerve action potentials (SNAPs); the findings were not diagnostic of demyelinating neuropathy. Two years later however, more prominent findings of primary demyelination appeared on repeat studies. There was evidence of clinical deterioration with a decline in walking, mild weakness of his interosseous muscles, and weakness of toe dorsiflexors. His sensory loss had advanced. He had temporal dispersion in his ulnar motor territory, a lengthening of his peroneal distal motor latency with a fall in the peroneal motor conduction velocity [Table 9.1 and Figure 9.1]. Denervation was identified in the tibialis anterior (fibrillations, positive sharp waves, and fasciculations). A course of intravenous gamma globulin (IVIG) was associated with improved electrophysiological results but produced relatively little symptomatic improvement. Upon returning to the country and clinic after a 2-year absence, he showed further deterioration. Trials of prednisone, intravenous methylprednisolone, and azathioprine were associated with uncertain benefit and were complicated by out of country absences from follow-up and by the patient's intermittent decisions to stop treatments. Overall treatment was sporadic. Over the years of follow-up, IVIG was associated with at least two documented episodes of clinical and electrophysiological improvement but the patient declined

Table 9.1. Serial electrophysiological studies (selected)

| Date | Ulnar* | | | Peroneal† | | | Comment |
	CMAPd	CMAPp	CV	CMAPd	CMAPp	CV	
1994	8.7	5.8	44	3.2	3.3	39	
1996	**5.2**	**3.8**	**49**	**0.89**	**0.71**	**33**	
1996	10.6	7.7	46	1.7	1.4	30	**Post-IVIG**
1998	9.2	6.1	44	1.7	1.2	28	IVIG, prednisone
2000	7.1	5.0	45	0.12	0.07	29	No therapy
2001	**8.7**	**7.3**	**41**	**0.31**	**0.24**	**29**	**Azathioprine, IVIG**
2006	7.7	5.6	34	0.02			No therapy
2007	5.3	3.4	33	abs	abs		Refused therapy

* Studies were done at wrist, below and above elbow (and higher), but above elbow results not shown.
† Studies were done at ankle, fibular head, and knee but knee results not shown; absent SNAPs were noted in all studies in the median, ulnar, sural, and superficial peroneal territories; median and tibial studies not shown.
CVs: conduction velocity [m/s] in the forearm segment (ulnar) or below the knee (peroneal) (normal, >50 in ulnar, 40 in peroneal); CMAP: compound muscle action potential (d = distal; p = proximal (mV); normal, >5.0 ulnar, 2.0 peroneal).

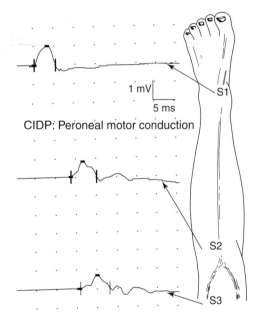

Figure 9.1 Examples of peroneal motor waveforms in the patient described in this vignette. The CMAPs (compound muscle action potentials) illustrated were recorded from the extensor digitorum brevis with stimulation at the ankle (S1), fibular head (S2), and knee (S3). Note that the CMAP amplitudes are reduced (normal, >2.0 mV) and dispersed on more proximal stimulation.

was wheelchair bound. Sphincter function remained intact. His electrophysiological studies showed loss or absence of motor potentials with dispersion, slowing of conduction velocity, and diffuse loss of SNAPs. Compared with his original studies, his upper limb CMAPs had declined by over 50% and his lower limb CMAPs had disappeared [Table 9.1]. Throughout his course, neuropathic pain was a significant and unrelenting problem. He was admitted twice to the Neurology Unit but became noncompliant and refused rehabilitation, immunomodulatory therapy, psychiatric input, or an assessment by the pain service.

CSF identified an elevated protein (0.87 g/L), normal glucose, and no white cells. A gastrocnemius muscle biopsy early in his course showed scattered atrophic fibers and rare grouped fibers. A sural nerve biopsy performed before his evaluation in our clinic identified loss of large myelinated axons, axonal degeneration, macrophage infiltration, and thin fibers with some evidence of segmental demyelination. Inflammation or onion bulbs were not identified. Amyloid was not present. The overall pathological diagnosis was that of CIDP. He declined further nerve biopsies to help substantiate the diagnosis, given his difficulties with treatment regimens. The evolution of his course and his electrophysiology results however, clarified the diagnosis.

Other investigations were either normal or negative and included: complete blood count, glucose, electrolytes, creatinine, uric acid, calcium, albumin, phosphorus, CK, LDH, bilirubin, alkaline phosphatase,

further treatment. Fourteen years after his original presentation to our clinic, he exhibited substantial deterioration with diffuse limb weakness especially distally (bilateral foot drop), distal wasting, arreflexia, and loss of sensation distal to his knees and elbows. He

ALT, GGT, ESR, TSH, B12 level, red cell folate, RPR (syphilis serology), HIV serology, serum protein electrophoresis (repeated assays), ANA, SS-A/Ro, anti-DNA, rheumatoid factor, antibodies to GM1, MAG (courtesy of Pestronk lab, Washington University), anti-Yo, anti-Hu, anti-MPP-1 and antibodies to Purkinje cells, 24-h Holter monitor, CT head scan, CT angiogram of brain, CT abdomen and pelvis, brain MRI. His cholesterol level was mildly elevated (7.33 mmol/L; normal, <6.2). An ECG suggested mild right ventricular hypertrophy. An MRI of the cervical intraspinal space showed multilevel degenerative disc disease without root or cord compression.

Pain description

In his initial clinic visit, the patient described cramps in his limbs and prickling, burning sensations below his knees particularly in the feet and posterior calves, and in his forearms. Over his course, he used a large number of medications for pain including diazepam, acetaminophen with codeine, gabapentin (up to 2700 mg/day was unhelpful), cesamet, oxycontin, capsaicin cream, amitriptyline, meperidine, morphine, hydromorphone, and nortriptyline. Their benefits were uncertain because of highly variable follow-up and compliance. Several regimens were stopped on his own without a clear report of the reasons or results of their use. He had noticed partial benefit with amitriptyline (50–75 mg qhs) but discontinued the medication. Long-acting morphine sulfate (MS contin 30 mg twice daily) provided some relief but unfortunately, the patient also developed opioid-related confusion and somnolence. He continued to report intense and unremitting pain in his legs below the knees and forearms. It was unclear whether immunomodulatory therapy (IVIG, prednisone), given intermittently during his course, helped with pain relief.

Discussion

This patient had a progressive, eventually severe motor and sensory polyneuropathy with prominent neuropathic pain. He had at least two remissions in his clinical condition when successful sustained immunotherapy (IVIG, prednisone and IVIG) was administered. Unfortunately depression, noncompliance, and long absences from clinic made it difficult to optimize either his immunotherapy or his neuropathic pain medication. By the time of his final hospitalization when he refused all treatment, he manifested essentially untreated and severe CIDP rendering him near bed bound with encephalopathic complications of opioid use.

The diagnosis of CIDP is confirmed by the clinical findings of a progressive or recurrent motor and sensory polyneuropathy, electrophysiological findings of primary demyelination (prolonged distal motor latencies, conduction slowing, conduction block, temporal dispersion, and prolonged F wave latencies), features of primary demyelination on nerve biopsy (segmental or paranodal demyelination with or without inflammation), and rises in CSF protein without a pleocytosis. Although they were not evident during early evaluations, our patient eventually displayed all of these findings. He fulfilled strict diagnostic criteria for CIDP as originally delineated by the American Academy of Neurology (1) and more recent criteria by the European Federation of Neurological Societies/Peripheral Nerve Society (2). CIDP is described as relapsing in approximately 65% of patients and as progressive in 35% of patients (3). Our patient was typical of the latter group.

Other features of CIDP that suggest axon loss include loss of motor and sensory potentials and denervation (fibrillations and positive sharp waves) on electrophysiological testing. Similarly nerve biopsies may show prominent axon loss. Our patient exhibited these findings.

Prednisone, azathioprine, plasma exchange, and IVIG all have an evidence basis for their use in CIDP. Randomized trials however, have largely been limited to short-term management of CIDP patients and consequently, long-term descriptions of the fate of these patients are rare. They include instances of rapid neurological deterioration. Some patients do not respond to therapy (up to a third in some trials) despite a firm diagnosis of CIDP. Two important neuropathies to consider in the differential diagnosis of CIDP are inherited sensitivity to pressure palsy (HNPP), an autosomal dominant disorder with a mutation in myelin protein PMP22, and sporadic or inherited amyloidosis with late onset. A family history of entrapment neuropathies in HNPPP may not always be forthcoming. Amyloidosis is usually progressive as an exclusive axonal disorder, but some cases may have features of primary demyelination (4). Our patient did not have a family history of neuropathy, entrapment at sites of compression, a monoclonal protein, or neuropathic ulcers. Amyloid was not identified in his muscle or nerve biopsy.

Pain in CIDP

Neuropathic pain as a complication of CIDP is thought less common than in other forms of neuropathy. McCombe et al. (3) reported pain, ranging from burning feet to aching muscle pain, as a chief complaint in 20% of patients; our patient experienced these symptoms as well. Toth and Au (5) reported neuropathic pain in 41% of patients with immune mediated polyneuropathy. In previous work, we described two patients with prominent upper limb neuropathic pain complicating CIDP (6). Clinical and electrophysiological worsening was associated with deep and distressing upper limb aching. In one patient, discomfort regularly predicted electrophysiological relapse of his neuropathy before the onset of more obvious clinical signs. Resolution of the pain also predicted improvement. Boukhris et al. (7) examined 5 of 27 patients with CIDP that had chronic progressive disease and prominent pain, similar to our cases. Bilateral radicular-like pain in three patients, paresthesiae in four patients, and lower limb involvement in three patients were described. As in other CIDP patients without pain, these patients had clinical, electrophysiological, and biopsy features of demyelinating neuropathy. Using a visual analog scale, the pain intensity was rated as 9/10 pretreatment and 4/10 after treatment combining analgesic agents with immunomodulatory therapy.

It is interesting to speculate why pain may be a feature of CIDP. Compression secondary to nerve root hypertrophy is a possible explanation. Another is the generation of ectopic axonal discharges from axons exposed to low grade chronic inflammation, the mediators described in other chapters of this text. Finally, loss of large fiber input at the level of the dorsal horn may contribute to undampened pain neurotransmission. Our patient highlighted the intensive pain and immunomodulatory care required for some CIDP patients, made particularly problematic when compliance and follow-up are compromised.

References

(1) Ad Hoc Subcommittee of the American Academy of Neurology AIDS Taskforce. Research criteria for diagnosis of chronic inflammatory demyelinating polyneuropathy (CIDP). *Neurology* 1991;41:617–618.

(2) European Federation of Neurological Societies/ Peripheral Nerve Society Guideline on management of chronic inflammatory demyelinating polyradiculoneuropathy. Report of a joint task force of the European Federation of Neurological Societies and the Peripheral Nerve Society. *J Peripher Nerv Syst* 2005;10:220–228.

(3) McCombe PA, Pollard JD, McLeod JG. Chronic inflammatory demyelinating polyradiculoneuropathy. A clinical and electrophysiological study of 92 cases. *Brain* 1987;110:1617–1630.

(4) Benson MD, Kincaid JC. The molecular biology and clinical features of amyloid neuropathy. *Muscle Nerve* 2007;36:411–423.

(5) Toth C, Au S. A prospective identification of neuropathic pain in specific chronic polyneuropathy syndromes and response to pharmacological therapy. *Pain* 2008;138:657–666.

(6) Zochodne DW, Brunet DG. Upper limb pain in chronic demyelinating polyneuropathy: electrophysiological correlates. *Acta Neurol Scand* 1994;90:270–275.

(7) Boukhris S, Magy L, Khalil M, Sindou P, Vallat JM. Pain as the presenting symptom of chronic inflammatory demyelinating polyradiculoneuropathy (CIDP). *J Neurol Sci* 2007;254:33–38.

Chapter

10

Pain and diabetic polyneuropathy (DPN)

Diabetic polyneuropathy (DPN) is one of the most common causes of neuropathic pain. Pain may be the presenting feature of DPN, and it may be severe despite relatively modest evidence of peripheral nerve damage. Diabetes mellitus (DM) can be associated with several forms of neuropathy, or nerve damage, including focal neuropathies such as carpal tunnel syndrome and lumbosacral plexopathy. In this case we emphasize DPN, a generalized form of neuropathy that can be diagnosed in up to 50% of diabetic patients, but we also highlight how it can accompany focal neuropathies in the same patient. We describe a type 2 diabetic patient who developed severe and painful DPN associated with poor compliance with his diabetes treatment regimen.

Clinical case vignette

A 58-year-old right-handed man had a 3-year history of type 2 DM, on treatment with glyburide, with poor compliance of blood glucose monitoring and reluctance to attend specific diabetes education clinics. Randomly sampled blood glucose levels taken by his daughter ranged from 16 to 31 mmol/L. There was no history of nephropathy or retinopathy when he presented with neuropathic symptoms.

He described a feeling of "pads" on the soles of his feet for approximately 1 year that sometimes interfered with his balance. He denied pain, loss of sensation, or paresthesiae on initial visits to the neurology clinic. He also denied weakness of his muscles or loss of balance otherwise. Erectile dysfunction had been present for 1 year, but he had no other autonomic nervous system symptoms beyond rare dizziness with standing. He had previously been healthy. There was a family history of DM involving his father and two brothers.

On initial neurological examination, he had intact mental functioning beyond denial of his medical problems, with normal speech and cranial nerves. He had

wasting of ulnar innervated hand muscles and extensor digitorum brevis muscles with weakness in his ulnar hand muscles (Grade 4/5 MRC) and toe dorsiflexors (4+/5). He had diffuse loss of deep tendon reflexes. Sensation to pinprick and light touch was impaired in the distal legs and feet, and there was analgesia and anesthesia in his toes. Vibration perception was absent in his toes and position sensitivity was normal. He had difficulty walking tandem or standing on his heels. There was no Romberg's sign. There were no foot ulcers. There was a 25 mm Hg drop in his systolic blood pressure with standing. His overall findings indicated moderately severe DPN with autonomic involvement and superimposed bilateral focal ulnar neuropathies.

Electrophysiological studies identified prolonged upper limb distal motor latencies, slowing of motor conduction velocities, and low amplitude CMAPs in the median and ulnar nerves. There was temporal dispersion in the ulnar motor territory. Only very small amplitude distal tibial CMAPs over abductor hallucis could be recorded with prolonged distal latencies. The peroneal CMAPs recorded over extensor digitorum brevis muscles were absent. He had complete absence of upper and lower limb sensory potentials in the median, ulnar, radial, superficial peroneal, and sural nerves. Needle electromyography identified fibrillation potentials and positive sharp waves in the tibialis anterior and first dorsal interosseous muscles with a reduced number of enlarged, rapidly firing voluntary motor unit potentials. Overall, the findings indicated a severe motor and sensory polyneuropathy with prominent features of axonal degeneration and superimposed features of primary demyelination. These electrophysiological abnormalities were more severe than the clinical findings or the history had suggested.

Other laboratory investigations were normal (negative), including complete blood count, alkaline phosphatase, ALT, creatinine, urinalysis, serum protein electrophoresis, ESR, and TSH. His cholesterol was elevated at 5.34 mmol/L (normal, <5.20) with normal triglycerides and HDL, and elevated LDL at 3.75 mmol/L (normal, <3.40). Fasting glucose was 13.2 mmol/L and hemoglobin A1C was 0.091 (normal, <0.061). His CK level was mildly elevated at 490 (normal, <195 U/L).

Over the next 1–2 years, there was marginal improvement in his compliance and a consultation with a diabetologist was arranged. Signs of his DPN continued to progress with bilateral foot drop, sensory loss in his hands and distal to his knees, and a Romberg sign. He would stumble on rough terrain at work. By year 2 after diagnosis, he had developed prominent lower limb pain. Gabapentin and ankle/foot orthoses were prescribed. Four years after his original visit to the Neurology clinic he required treatment for a small preulcerative lesion on the skin in the second right PIP joint and fifth metatarsal head area.

Pain description

At 6 years after his initial visit (9 years from diagnosis of DM), he described pain in his calves and thighs worse with resting after activity. Pain interfered with his ability to sleep. It was aggravated by cold contact and included a tingling component but its most common descriptor was aching discomfort rather than burning or squeezing. His pain was continuous and he ranked it as severe as 8/10. He experienced some benefit from gabapentin, did not tolerate pregabalin or amitriptyline, and was also treated with low-dose, long-acting morphine (15 mg q12h).

Discussion

This patient developed a relentlessly progressive form of DPN in the setting of very poor control of his type 2 DM. Prominent early features were loss of sensation and focal ulnar neuropathies, later pain, skin ulceration, and finally, progressive distal motor weakness in the legs. The electrophysiological features identified prominent axonal loss but also features of primary demyelination, both well recognized in advanced DPN. In the setting of uncontrolled hyperglycemia, his DPN progressed over 6 years of follow-up. Gabapentin provided only partial pain control and eventually, the patient required a low-dose opioid. Progresssive sensory alterations in DPN are illustrated in Figure 10.1.

Pain in DPN

Pain can develop at any stage of DPN. Symptoms may include nocturnal burning discomfort, allodynia, electrical jolts, but also deep aching pain, as described by our patient. In some patients, there is prominent pain before signs of polyneuropathy develop. In the absence of frank axon loss, this indicates that altered excitability, associated with early molecular changes of axons and sensory neurons in ganglia, may be responsible.

Several mechanisms have been considered in the pathogenesis of neuropathic pain in DPN. The literature addressing neuropathic pain in animal models of disease has rapidly expanded over the past decade. Abnormalities that develop in diabetic peripheral neurons include changes in the distributions of sodium or calcium channels that favor the generation of abnormal ectopic discharges and initiate the pain cascade. In particular, the specific channels linked to experimental DPN include $Ca_v3.2$ T-type calcium channels (upregulation) (1), sodium channels $Na_v1.3$ (upregulation), $Na_v1.7$ (upregulation, increased tyrosine phosphorylation), $Na_v1.6$ and $Na_v1.8$ (both downregulated but with increased serine/threonine phosphorylation; $Na_v1.6$ also had increased tyrosine phosphorylation) (2); $Na_v1.9$ (upregulated) and β3 (upregulated) (3, 4).

There is however, considerable variability amid the results and conclusions in the experimental work. Three major test paradigms are routinely used to evaluate pain in experimental DPN models. These include the latency of withdrawal to a thermal stimulus applied to the hindpaw (Hargreaves test) (5), the response to mechanical stimulation of the hindpaw with either a von-Frey hair of graded bending strength or an electronically controlled probe of defined force (Randall-Selitto test) and the latency to tailflick withdrawal to a heat stimulus applied to the tail. Yet another approach is to superimpose the hindpaw formalin injection paradigm on diabetic models. This model generates two phases of pain behavior, with the second exaggerated in diabetic models (6). Calcutt (7) has reviewed some of the difficulties in analyzing models of neuropathic pain, citing various technical variations and inconsistencies. For example, a thermal stimulus applied to a rat paw may penetrate more deeply and trigger afferent responses from deeper sensory axons than discrete mechanical stimuli. An important consideration in DPN pain models is the duration of diabetes. In outbred Swiss-Webster mice studied serially over several months of diabetes, initial

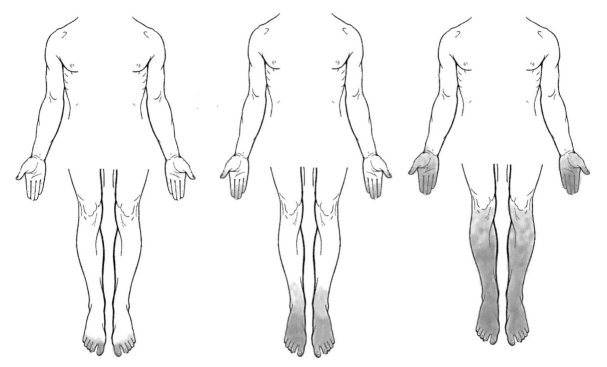

Figure 10.1. Progressive stocking then stocking and glove sensory changes in a patient with diabetic polyneuropathy. The shaded areas can represent pain, paresthesiae, or loss of sensation. Reproduced with permission from *Diabetic Neurology* (23).

thermal hyperalgesia and mechanical allodynia were later followed by loss of thermal and mechanical sensation, consistent with eventual loss of distal skin innervation as neuropathy progressed (8).

Changes of specific ion channel molecular subclasses may develop in DPN and account for different types of pain syndromes. For example, in some models including analysis of ZDF diabetic rats, a model of type 2 diabetes mellitus, mechanical allodynia was more prominent than thermal hyperalgesia (9–11). While the technical factors discussed above may account for these differences, recent literature indicates for example that N-type calcium channel splice variant isoforms labelled e37a and 337b (12) mediate different forms of pain. Similarly, A-type potassium channels attenuate mechanical but not thermal hyperalgesia (see Chapter 1).

Recent work by Chattopadhyay et al. (13) demonstrated that rats with STZ-induced diabetes of duration 6 weeks upregulate $Na_v1.7$ channels in DRGs and that a subcutaneous inoculation of a herpes simplex-based vector expressing proenkephalin reversed these changes. At the same time, heat and cold hyperalgesia and mechanical allodynia were reversed. The authors further argued that a high concentration of glucose (45 mmol/L) could itself induce rises in the $Na_v1.7$ in neonatal rat sensory neurons through the actions of phosphorylated PKC and p38. Dobretsov et al. (14) argue instead that impaired insulin signaling before frank diabetes, instead of hyperglycemia, is responsible for the dysfunction of sensory axons.

Other mechanisms of neuropathic pain specifically in the setting of diabetes have been investigated. A bradykinin B1 receptor (BKB1-R) antagonist reversed thermal hyperalgesia in two type 1 diabetic models in rats: STZ diabetic and BB/Wor-DP rats (15). Hong and Wiley demonstrated that painful experimental diabetic neuropathy was associated with changes in the expression of the VR1 (vanilloid, TRPV1) receptor (rises in large neurons, declines in small neurons). Rises in the tetrameric membrane-expressed version of the TRPV1 receptor during experimental diabetes were also linked to rises in its sensitivity through PKC-mediated phosphorylation. PKC has been linked to the development of pain in models of DPN. For example, inhibition of PKC also attenuated hyperalgesia in STZ diabetic rats (16), whereas activation of PKC increased thermal hyperalgesia (17). Finally, changes at the level

47

of the dorsal horn of the spinal cord or higher may also be implicated in the development of neuropathic pain (18, 19). Specifically Ramos et al. (19) show that rats with early STZ-induced diabetes had rises in spinal COX-2 protein and activity that accompanied abnormalities in pain behavior with formalin testing. Hyperalgesia to formalin and rises in COX-2 were prevented by insulin treatment or by using an aldose reductase inhibitor capable of crossing the blood–brain barrier to act on the dorsal horn of the spinal cord. Overall, these findings indicate that DPN is associated with multilevel changes in the neuraxis that promote pain, including alterations of primary sensory neurons and abnormal signaling through the dorsal horn of the spinal cord.

The current state of the literature evaluating analgesic therapy for human diabetic polyneuropathy has been reviewed elsewhere and is considered in Chapter 32 (20, 21). Briefly, there is evidence for the use of tricyclic antidepressants, gabapentin, pregabalin, opioids (including tramadol), and duloxetine. Opioids and gabapentin may have synergistic actions (22). In complex diabetic patients with renal disease and involvement of other organ systems, gabapentin or opioids may be the safest agents of choice. Gabapentin dosage requires downward revision in renal failure patients but it remains effective. Initial therapy with gabapentin is one of the authors' (DZ) treatment of first choice, perhaps beginning with a low evening dose (e.g., 300 mg). Side-effects include cognitive dysfunction and dizziness particularly with the highest doses used (4000 mg). Opioids also cause cognitive dysfunction and constipation.

References

(1) Jagodic MM, Pathirathna S, Nelson MT, et al. Cell-specific alterations of T-type calcium current in painful diabetic neuropathy enhance excitability of sensory neurons. *J Neurosci* 2007;27:3305–3316.

(2) Hong S, Morrow TJ, Paulson PE, Isom LL, Wiley JW. Early painful diabetic neuropathy is associated with differential changes in tetrodotoxin-sensitive and -resistant sodium channels in dorsal root ganglion neurons in the rat. *J Biol Chem* 2004;279:29341–29350.

(3) Craner MJ, Klein JP, Renganathan M, Black JA, Waxman SG. Changes of sodium channel expression in experimental painful diabetic neuropathy. *Ann Neurol* 2002;52:786–792.

(4) Shah BS, Gonzalez MI, Bramwell S, Pinnock RD, Lee K, Dixon AK. Beta3, a novel auxiliary subunit for the voltage gated sodium channel is upregulated in sensory neurones following streptozocin induced diabetic neuropathy in rat. *Neurosci Lett* 2001;309:1–4.

(5) Hargreaves K, Dubner R, Brown F, Flores C, Joris J. A new and sensitive method for measuring thermal nociception in cutaneous hyperalgesia. *Pain* 1988;32:77–88.

(6) Calcutt NA, Jorge MC, Yaksh TL, Chaplan SR. Tactile allodynia and formalin hyperalgesia in streptozotocin-diabetic rats: effects of insulin, aldose reductase inhibition and lidocaine. *Pain* 1996;68:293–299.

(7) Calcutt NA. Experimental models of painful diabetic neuropathy. *J Neurol Sci* 2004;220:137–139.

(8) Toth C, Rong LL, Yang C, et al. RAGE and experimental diabetic neuropathy. *Diabetes* 2008;57:1002–1017.

(9) Brussee V, Guo GF, Dong YY, et al. Distal degenerative sensory neuropathy in a long term type 2 diabetes rat model. *Diabetes* 2008;57:1664–1673.

(10) Fox A, Eastwood C, Gentry C, Manning D, Urban L. Critical evaluation of the streptozotocin model of painful diabetic neuropathy in the rat. *Pain* 1999;81:307–316.

(11) Romanovsky D, Cruz NF, Dienel GA, Dobretsov M. Mechanical hyperalgesia correlates with insulin deficiency in normoglycemic streptozotocin-treated rats. *Neurobiol Dis* 2006;24:384–394.

(12) Altier C, Dale CS, Kisilevsky AE, et al. Differential role of N-type calcium channel splice isoforms in pain. *J Neurosci* 2007;27:6363–6373.

(13) Chattopadhyay M, Mata M, Fink DJ. Continuous delta-opioid receptor activation reduces neuronal voltage-gated sodium channel (NaV1.7) levels through activation of protein kinase C in painful diabetic neuropathy. *J Neurosci* 2008;28:6652–6658.

(14) Dobretsov M, Ghaleb AH, Romanovsky D, Pablo CS, Stimers JR. Impaired insulin signaling as a potential trigger of pain in diabetes and prediabetes. *Int Anesthesiol Clin* 2007;45:95–105.

(15) Gabra BH, Benrezzak O, Pheng LH, et al. Inhibition of type 1 diabetic hyperalgesia in streptozotocin-induced Wistar versus spontaneous gene-prone BB/Worchester rats: efficacy of a selective bradykinin B1 receptor antagonist. *J Neuropathol Exp Neurol* 2005;64:782–789.

(16) Ahlgren SC, Levine JD. Protein kinase C inhibitors decrease hyperalgesia and C-fiber hyperexcitability in

the streptozotocin-diabetic rat. *J Neurophysiol* 1994;72:684–692.

(17) Ohsawa M, Kamei J. Possible involvement of spinal protein kinase C in thermal allodynia and hyperalgesia in diabetic mice. *Eur J Pharmacol* 1999;372:221–228.

(18) Calcutt NA. Potential mechanisms of neuropathic pain in diabetes. *Int Rev Neurobiol* 2002;50: 205–228.

(19) Ramos KM, Jiang Y, Svensson CI, Calcutt NA. Pathogenesis of spinally mediated hyperalgesia in diabetes. *Diabetes* 2007;56:1569–1576.

(20) Zochodne DW. Diabetes mellitus and the peripheral nervous system: manifestations and mechanisms. *Muscle Nerve* 2007;36:144–166.

(21) Vinik A. Clinical review: use of antiepileptic drugs in the treatment of chronic painful diabetic neuropathy. *J Clin Endocrinol Metab* 2005;90:4936–4945.

(22) Gilron I, Bailey JM, Tu D, Holden RR, Weaver DF, Houlden RL. Morphine, gabapentin, or their combination for neuropathic pain. *N Engl J Med* 2005;352:1324–1334.

(23) Zochodne DW, Kline GA, Smith E, Hill MD. *Diabetic Neurology*. New York: Informa, 2010.

Chapter

11

Painful idiopathic polyneuropathy

A large proportion of polyneuropathies, especially sensory polyneuropathies, are classified as idiopathic because their specific etiologies have not been identified. Although additional causes of polyneuropathy have emerged within this group, the proportion with an unknown cause remains substantial. Some are associated with glucose intolerance. In this case, we describe a patient with a painful idiopathic sensory polyneuropathy followed over 7 years. Pharmacotherapy was challenging because of associated side-effects. Whereas several comorbid conditions were present, none were identified as causing the condition.

Clinical case vignette

A 70-year-old right-handed retired professor was evaluated for a 10-year history of sensory symptoms in his legs. The onset was gradual, and the symptoms had been progressive. He described loss of balance and symmetrical burning pain in his legs, soles of his feet, and toes. His legs felt heavy and "leaden." There were sensations of tingling and numbness in his fingers. There was loss of sensation in his legs distal to the knees, but he denied specific muscle weakness. As a result, he was no longer able to walk his dogs and had gained 30 lbs from inactivity. There was no history of foot ulcer. He noticed constipation and bladder urgency. While gabapentin provided some relief, he was unable to increase the dose beyond 1200 mg daily because of lower limb swelling.

His prior medical history was complex with osteoarthritis requiring a previous left knee and right hip replacement. Other problems included chronic neck and back discomfort, hypertension, dyslipidemia, sleep apnea, benign prostatic hypertrophy, gastroesophageal reflux, chronic hearing loss attributed to military service and working in a mine, and a previous TIA. He had prior diverticulitis surgery, tonsillectomy, and a breast reduction. Medications included candesartan, amiloride, omeprazole, celecoxib, allo-

purinol, gabapentin, trazodone, and quinine sulfate. He used 2 ounces of ethanol weekly and was a nonsmoker. There was no family history of neurological disease.

On his initial neurological examination, he had stocking loss of sensation to his knees and loss in his volar fingers involving light touch and pinprick. There was analgesia in his toes without anesthesia. He had absent vibration sensation in one large toe and reduced vibration sensation in the other. Position sensation was normal. Motor power and tone were normal throughout and there was no wasting excepting the extensor digitorum brevis muscles. Ankle reflexes were absent. His gait was antalgic. He had a mild intention tremor. There was no Romberg sign. General examination identified obesity, distal foot swelling, and changes of osteoarthritis in his knees.

Investigations included the following normal studies: complete blood count, ESR, calcium, serum and urine protein electrophoresis, electrolytes, creatinine, TSH, B12, fasting and 2-h PC glucose, hemoglobin A1C, ANA, and GGT. A methylmalonic acid level was borderline elevated (0.20 μM; normal, 0.02–0.15). Imaging studies of the lumbar spine identified changes of spondylosis, L45 foraminal stenosis, but no spinal stenosis. Cervical MRI identified spondylosis and mild spinal stenosis. Electrophysiological testing identified low amplitude distal peroneal CMAPs, borderline reductions in motor conduction velocities in his legs, an absent superficial peroneal sensory potential, and a low amplitude sural potential. In the upper limbs, motor conduction was normal, but sensory potentials were reduced in amplitude or absent. Needle electromyography identified occasional fibrillation potentials in his tibialis anterior muscle with reduced numbers of enlarged motor unit potentials. Gastrocnemius had enlarged motor unit potentials. Right first dorsal interosseous and deltoid muscles were normal. A second set of studies 2 years later identified further declines in his lower limb CMAPs,

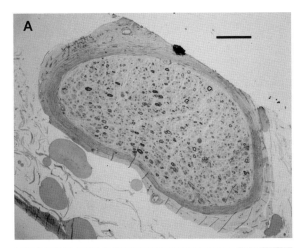

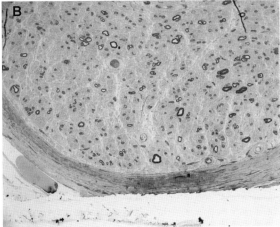

(**Figure 11.1.** Transverse sections of sural nerve biopsy from the patient described in this vignette. The sample is epon-embedded and stained with toluidine blue at lower power (A) and higher power (B) [Bar = 50 μm for A and 100 μm for B]. Note the severe and widespread diffuse loss of large and small myelinated axons. Occasional myelinated fibers are clustered indicating regenerative sprouts.

and his sural potential had disappeared. A right sural nerve biopsy identified severe loss of myelinated axons (>90%), mild signs of active axonal degeneration without inflammation, vascular changes, or amyloid deposition. Occasional regenerative clusters and occasional thinly myelinated axons were identified [Figure 11.1].

The patient was followed intermittently for 7 years. Pregabalin caused unacceptable lower limb swelling. At the age of 74 and following a trial of nabilone prescribed by the pain clinic, he developed tachycardia and at the same time suffered a left parietal cerebral infarct from which he made a near complete recovery. Long-acting codeine and oxycontin caused nausea.

Topiramate was associated with nausea and dizziness. He continued taking gabapentin in varying doses (up to 3900 mg) but was uncertain of its benefit. He noticed some benefit from hydromorphone and dimenhydrinate combined and from the use of TENS (transcutaneous electrical nerve stimulation). Venlafaxine had uncertain benefit. By age 81, he had ongoing loss of sensation to light touch and pinprick below his knees, absent vibration sensation in his toes, and loss of all deep tendon reflexes excepting the left triceps. Motor function was preserved. He had stopped his opioid medication and had decided against further specific neuropathic pain medications.

Pain description

The patient experienced continuous burning lower limb pain below the knees involving his soles and toes. He had a sensation "like sandpaper" over his feet. Other descriptors included squeezing, pressure, tingling, "pins and needles," and stabbing, but he denied allodynia from touching or cold. He generally rated the pain intensity as 4/10 on average, and in a range of 3–5/10; his ability to sleep was impacted. On some visits, he rated the pain intensity somewhat higher at 8/10. The pain had a major impact on his ability to enjoy life. He rated his health state as 2/10, with 10 representing the best imaginable health state.

Discussion

The largest category of painful small fiber peripheral neuropathies are idiopathic, or of uncertain cause (1–3). This overlaps with patients classified as having chronic idiopathic axonal polyneuropathy, thought to constitute approximately 10–18% of patients with chronic axonal polyneuropathy (4–7). These series describe the mean age of onset as 57, not unlike the onset at age 60 in our patient. Our patient's neuropathy was not strictly small fiber given his symptom of imbalance and the detection of reduced vibration perception and loss of deep tendon reflexes. In addition, his lower limb sensory nerve action potentials gradually declined over time. His diagnosis was likely best classified as mixed fiber neuropathy. In patients without signs of large fiber involvement and normal nerve conduction studies, skin biopsy may identify loss of epidermal axons, indicating small fiber involvement. An extensive investigation in our patient, including nerve biopsy, failed to identify the cause, and his condition slowly progressed over time. Repeated tests for impaired glucose metabolism or diabetes mellitus were negative, and he did not use significant amounts of ethanol. A skin biopsy was not performed. Our patient resembles those described by Notermans et al. (8) who followed 75 patients with chronic idiopathic axonal polyneuropathy over 5 years and only discovered a definite cause in four patients (two inherited, one CIDP, and one secondary to alcohol).

Hughes et al. (6) studied 50 consecutive patients with chronic idiopathic axonal polyneuropathy and compared them to 50 control persons from the same region. Twenty-two patients (44%) had pain and 26 (52%) had evidence of only sensory involvement. There was no increased risk of ethanol use, impaired glucose tolerance, or fasting hyperglycemia in the patients with polyneuropathy. Elevated triglyceride levels had a significant association with polyneuropathy. Patients with chronic idiopathic axonal polyneuropathy were more likely to be older men, and the features were gradually progressive and symmetric. Autonomic symptoms were not prominent.

Despite the failure of Hughes et al. to link chronic idiopathic axonal polyneuropathy to impaired glucose metabolism, other series have identified a linkage. Singleton et al. (9) reported on the records of 89 patients with idiopathic polyneuropathy and identified 28 (31%) with frank diabetes mellitus. Of the remaining 61 patients, 25% had impaired glucose tolerance, a prevalence of twice that expected in an unselected population. Approximately one third had neuropathic pain.

Nebuchennykh et al. (10) examined 70 patients from Norway with idiopathic sensory polyneuropathy. Sixteen patients (23%) had impaired glucose metabolism; 3% had frank diabetes mellitus, 4% had impaired fasting glucose, 3% had impaired fasting glucose and glucose tolerance and 13% had impaired glucose tolerance. Neuropathic pain was described in 69% of patients with impaired glucose metabolism and 68% of the remaining patients, indicating no significant difference in the predisposition to pain. Pure sensory involvement was present in 35% of those with impaired glucose metabolism and 48% of the remainder. Sural potentials were abnormal in 25% of those with impaired glucose metabolism and 13% of the remainder. Overall, the authors believed that the prevalence of impaired glucose metabolism was lower in the Norwegian population with neuropathy than in other reported series.

Bednarik et al. (11) evaluated 84 patients with painful sensory neuropathy and predominant small fiber involvement. In this study, individuals with signs of large fiber involvement were excluded, although they were included if they had abnormal sensory nerve conduction results. Thus, this group of patients differed from the patient reported here in our case vignette. Patients with motor involvement were also not included. In comparison to 47 asymptomatic age- and sex-matched control subjects, a multivariate regression model indicated that diabetes mellitus, chronic alcoholism, and serum cholesterol levels independently were associated with small fiber neuropathy. No etiology was identified in 22.6% of patients. Interestingly, the presence of sensory conduction changes, indicative of a more widespread spectrum of fiber involvement, did not influence the findings. Although not rigorously examined in this or other studies, we suspect that many strictly small fiber sensory neuropathies later develop involvement of larger fibers, as in our patient. Indeed, a significant proportion of patients initially diagnosed with exclusive sensory polyneuropathies may have subclinical motor abnormalities on electrophysiological testing (12). Our patient had wasted EDB muscles and low amplitude peroneal CMAPs without weakness.

Erdmann et al. (5) identified pain in 77% of the 56 patients they studied, among several other disabilities in patients with chronic idiopathic axonal polyneuropathy. Fatigue, loss of autonomy outdoors, and poor balance were also common among their group. Predictably, lower limbs had greater involvement, as might be expected, than the upper limbs.

Pain in chronic idiopathic axonal polyneuropathies

Despite differences among the series described above, neuropathic pain is a common and constant feature. Because the etiologies of many of these polyneuropathies remain unknown, the mechanisms of pain are unclear. In patients with impaired glucose tolerance, abnormalities of sensory neurons that generate pain may be similar to those secondary to frank diabetes (see Chapter 10). Recently, Faber et al. (13) identified mutations in the function of the sodium channel $Na_v1.7$ in a significant proportion of patients with idiopathic small fiber neuropathy. The SCN9A gene encodes for $Na_v1.7$, and the mutations resulted in a gain of function. As discussed in Chapter 1, pain syndromes including erythromelalgia and paroxysmal extreme pain disorder (PEPD) can arise from mutations of $Na_v1.7$ (14). Faber et al. studied 28 patients who met the strict criteria for idiopathic small fiber neuropathy: no underlying etiology, normal strength, normal tendon reflexes, normal vibration perception, and normal nerve conduction studies. The patients had reduced intraepidermal nerve fiber density plus abnormal quantitative sensory testing (QST) with at least two appropriate symptoms. Symptoms were burning feet, allodynia, diminished pain and/or temperature sensation, dry eyes or mouth, orthostatic dizziness, bowel and urinary disturbances, sweating abnormalities, visual accommodation problems or blurred vision, impotence, diminished ejaculation or lubrication, hot flashes, and palpitations. SCN9A analysis identified missense mutations in 8 of the 28 patients screened, rendering $Na_v1.7$ channels hyperexcitable. Overall, the group of patients with mutations was on average a younger population with a mean age of 32.4, making the suspicion of an inherited cause more likely. Pain was of distal onset and its intensity varied but it did not share the characteristics of temperature sensitivity observed in erythromelalgia. Seven of the 8 patients also had autonomic complaints. The authors suggested that abnormal sodium channel activation of small primary afferent fibers might lead to secondary degeneration and neuropathy.

Overall, the majority of patients with painful idiopathic polyneuropathies do not have an explanation for their symptoms. However, it may be that a range of additional ion channel changes, either primary or secondary, may eventually be linked to this condition.

References

(1) Periquet MI, Novak V, Collins MP, et al. Painful sensory neuropathy: prospective evaluation using skin biopsy. *Neurology* 1999;53:1641–1647.

(2) Lacomis D. Small-fiber neuropathy. *Muscle Nerve* 2002;26:173–188.

(3) Hoitsma E, Reulen JP, de BM, Drent M, Spaans F, Faber CG. Small fiber neuropathy: a common and important clinical disorder. *J Neurol Sci* 2004;227: 119–130.

(4) McLeod JG, Tuck RR, Pollard JD, Cameron J, Walsh JC. Chronic polyneuropathy of undetermined cause. *J Neurol Neurosurg Psychiatry* 1984;47:530–535.

(5) Erdmann PG, Teunissen LL, van Genderen FR, et al. Functioning of patients with chronic idiopathic axonal polyneuropathy (CIAP). *J Neurol* 2007;254: 1204–1211.

(6) Hughes RA, Umapathi T, Gray IA, et al. A controlled investigation of the cause of chronic idiopathic axonal polyneuropathy. *Brain* 2004;127:1723–1730.

(7) Dyck PJ, Oviatt KF, Lambert EH. Intensive evaluation of referred unclassified neuropathies yields improved diagnosis. *Ann Neurol* 1981;10:222–226.

(8) Notermans NC, Wokke JH, van der Graaf Y, Franssen H, van Dijk GW, Jennekens FG. Chronic idiopathic axonal polyneuropathy: a five year follow up. *J Neurol Neurosurg Psychiatry* 1994;57:1525–1527.

(9) Singleton JR, Smith AG, Bromberg MB. Painful sensory polyneuropathy associated with impaired glucose tolerance. *Muscle Nerve* 2001;24:1225–1228.

(10) Nebuchennykh M, Loseth S, Jorde R, Mellgren SI. Idiopathic polyneuropathy and impaired glucose metabolism in a Norwegian patient series. *Eur J Neurol* 2008;15:810–816.

(11) Bednarik J, Vlckova-Moravcova E, Bursova S, Belobradkova J, Dusek L, Sommer C. Etiology of small-fiber neuropathy. *J Peripher Nerv Syst* 2009;14:177–183.

(12) Chhibber S, Toth C. Lack of motor progression in isolated sensory peripheral neuropathy. *Can J Neurol Sci* 2010;37:517–520.

(13) Faber CG, Hoeijmakers JG, Ahn HS, et al. Gain of function Nav1.7 mutations in idiopathic small fiber neuropathy. *Ann Neurol* 2012;71:26–39.

(14) Cummins TR, Sheets PL, Waxman SG. The roles of sodium channels in nociception: Implications for mechanisms of pain. *Pain* 2007;131:243–257.

Chapter

12

Pain in vasculitic neuropathy

Neuropathy secondary to vasculitis, either systemic or confined to the peripheral nervous system, usually begins asymmetrically, classically as mononeuritis multiplex. Acute mononeuropathies from vasculitis may be very painful. A significant proportion of patients however, also present with a more symmetrical bilateral polyneuropathy secondary to underlying vasculitis. A patient with bilateral symmetric chronic neuropathy secondary to nonsystemic vasculitis is described.

Clinical case vignette

A 62-year-old recently widowed man presented with a 2-year history of burning pain and numbness of both lower legs, more pronounced on the left. After walking distances of more than 800 meters, both legs became painful. For longer walks, he used a cane because of a feeling of instability. He complained of brief episodes of spontaneous shooting pain in both legs that occurred approximately 10 times per day. At night, he suffered from frequent cramps in his calf muscles. Amitriptyline, taken as a nightly dose of 75 mg, provided no relief; higher doses were not tolerated because of micturition problems.

Examination revealed fasciculations in both calves, loss of achilles tendon reflexes, mild pareses of toe dorsiflexion, a stocking pattern of loss to all sensory qualities on both lower legs, and mild ataxia on standing. Nerve conduction studies gave normal results at the arms and showed moderate reduction of compound muscle action potential (CMAP) and sensory (SNAP) amplitudes in the tibial and sural nerves, respectively. Electromyography (EMG) of the lower leg muscles showed occasional fibrillations and fasciculations. Laboratory investigations including serum chemistry, complete blood count, erythrocyte sedimentation rate, serum vitamin B12 concentration, serum protein electrophoresis, antinuclear antibodies, anti-SSA/SSB antibodies, paraneoplastic antibodies,

rheumatoid factor, cryoglobulins, and serum complement were normal. Atypical anti-neutrophil cytoplasmic antibody (xANCA) was positive at 1:320. Cerebrospinal fluid showed mildly increased protein with 0.63 g/dl (normal, <0.45) and positive oligoclonal bands. Magnetic resonance tomography of the brain and spinal cord showed no indication of multiple sclerosis and no spinal stenosis. Sural nerve biopsy revealed a moderate axonal neuropathy with active axonal degeneration and perivascular inflammatory infiltrates, some of which infiltrated the vessel walls [Figure 12.1]. A tentative diagnosis of non-systemic vasculitic neuropathy (NSVN) was made and intravenous corticosteroids were given at a dose of 1 g/day for 3 consecutive days. The patient experienced rapid relief from the shooting pain, but painful nightly muscle cramps persisted. Magnesium substitution was not effective, and carbamazepine was initiated to reduce nerve hyperexcitability. Azathioprine, a steroid sparing agent, was added to the patient's medications; steroids were slowly tapered. It was discontinued 3 months later because of abdominal pain and vomiting. A second attempt to give azathioprine after the gastrointestinal symptoms had remitted led to rapid onset of the same symptoms. The drug was finally stopped after gastroscopy excluded other causes for his symptoms.

Four months later, the patient returned to the Neurology clinic with complaints of increased pain and reduced walking ability. He had bilateral foot drop and a markedly ataxic gait. His mood was subdued and he said that he did not enjoy life any more. Repeated high-dose steroids induced a second remission but symptoms returned once the steroids were tapered. Although carbamazepine provided sufficient relief from the nocturnal cramps, it was discontinued because of hyponatremia. Gabapentin was administered for neuropathic pain, and when required, an opioid (oxycodone) was added. This combination resulted in some relief and the patient rated his pain as bearable.

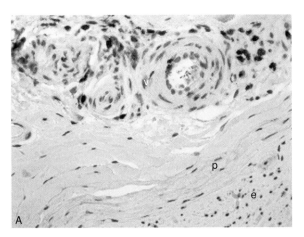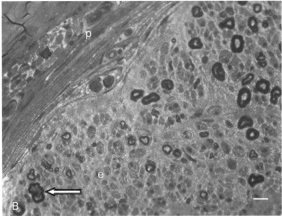

Figure 12.1 Photomicrographs of the patient's sural nerve biopsy. (A) Paraffin-embedded section immunoreacted for T lymphocytes with antibodies to CD3. Note perivascular T cells with occasional lymphocytes infiltrating the vessel wall. e = endoneurium, p = perineurium, v = vessels. (B) Semi-thin plastic-embedded section illustrating the enlarged and heavily vascularized perineurium (p), patchy nerve fiber loss in the endoneurium (e) and acute axonal degeneration (arrow). Bar = 10 μm.

The patient's symptoms were slowly progressive and eventually spread to the forearms. Over the next few years, several immunosuppressive treatment regimens were attempted. Cyclosporin A was given for a total of 9 months with gaps because of problems with the patient's health care provider. Several months after cyclosporine A was paused, the patient complained about progressive weakness of his fingers. On examination, mild weakness (MRC grade 4/5) of the finger extensors and abductors were seen bilaterally. Nerve conduction studies showed a deterioration of the tibial nerve territory CMAP. The patient required 10 mg of long-acting morphine daily for pain control. Over the next 2 years, the patient received additional courses of high-dose corticosteroids with identical results: abatement of symptoms that returned following tapering. Despite prophylaxis with calcium, vitamin D, and a bisphosphonate, osteoporosis had developed and back pain was an additional complaint. During a rehabilitation treatment, back pain worsened and the patient was admitted to hospital. X-ray of the lumbar spine showed a T12 compression fracture, which was confirmed on MRI and considered osteoporotic. Vertebroplasty was performed, resulting in almost complete relief of the back pain.

Gait ataxia was progressive. Repeated electrophysiological examinations showed a slow decline in motor nerve compound potential amplitudes [Figure 12.2]. Because the patient still complained of excruciating pain, the pain medication was changed to pregabalin and a fentanyl patch which finally brought relief. On one occasion soon after admission, the patient became somnolent due to opioid intoxication and was transferred to the intensive care unit. Drug toxicity was the result of self-medication with fentanyl patches for pain. The analgesic treatment was changed to a combination of pregabalin and amitriptyline. Muscle cramps were treated with quinidine. As before, the patient appeared to respond initially but experienced no long-term benefit. A course of intravenous immunoglobulin at a dose of 2 g/kg bodyweight was not effective. Finally, cyclophosphamide was initiated. Use of this drug had been avoided because systemic vasculitis had not been diagnosed and peripheral nerve vasculitis had not been fully confirmed despite the suggestive histological findings. The patient tolerated the drug well and received 12 cycles over the next year. Fortunately, the patient's condition stabilized under this treatment. Pain control was attained through a combination of pregabalin and tramadol. Muscle cramps were reduced with phenytoin, which was also tolerated well. On one occasion however, the patient developed an intercurrent infection and presented with blurred vision, nystagmus, and pronounced gait ataxia. Phenytoin blood levels had increased to 34.4 mg/L (therapeutic laboratory range, 5–10 mg/L). Symptoms rapidly settled after the drug was stopped and inflammatory parameters normalized. Oxcarbazepine, which was subsequently administered, also reduced the muscle cramps, but as with carbamazepine, led to severe hyponatremia; at a later stage, phenytoin was again prescribed and tolerated well by the patient. After

55

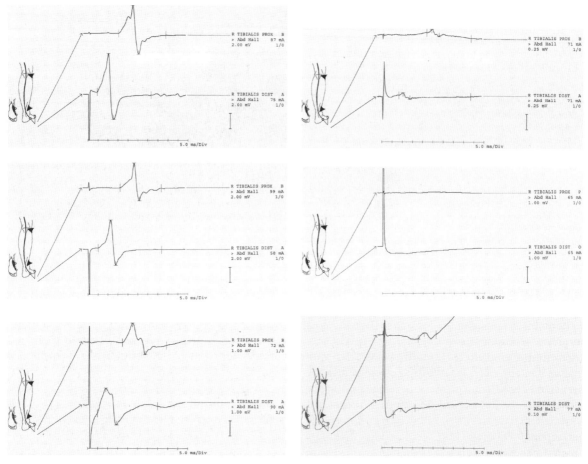

Figure 12.2 Evaluation of tibial nerve compound muscle action potential (CMAP) over time. Note slowly progressive reduction of CMAP amplitude, with the first signs of recovery in the last panel.

the 12th course of cyclophosphamide, the patient appeared stable and immunosuppression was stopped. Conversion to azathioprine was attempted, but as before, the patient experienced gastrointestinal side-effects. Six-month follow-up checks confirmed that the patient remained stable without the use of immuno-suppressive medication. When the patient was last seen, he had returned from a short vacation with his new partner. His mood was substantially improved, and he commented that his pain and his ataxia were alleviated "on the arm of his new love."

Pain description

This patient complained of different types of pain caused by at least three sets of pathological processes. Burning pain, numbness, and intermittent shooting pain in the lower legs were suggestive of a peripheral

neuropathy. Alternatively, a spinal lesion might have been responsible for these symptoms but this was not evident in the initial spinal MRI scans. Muscle cramps, mostly in the gastrocnemius and soleus muscle, were an early symptom and related to muscle denervation caused by the neuropathy. Back pain, which developed during the disease course, was caused by an osteo-porotic fracture. The patient had considerable diffi-culty describing the character or severity of his pain. Over the many years of his treatment, he refused to provide quantitative measures of pain. Instead, he used verbal descriptors for his pain, including "excruciat-ing," "unbearable," or "torturing."

Discussion

This patient's course was complicated by several fea-tures. The patient had various types and causes of pain due to several, ongoing pathological processes. He had typical neuropathic pain, with a combination of distally accentuated burning pain and numbness as well as intermittent shooting pain. The clinical and neurophysiological manifestations as described above confirmed this diagnosis (1). The patient also suffered from severe muscle cramps, which tended to persist even if the neuropathic pain was well controlled. Finally, he had a treatment-related complication; an osteoporotic fracture of the 12th thoracic vertebra also induced pain.

Several evidence-based guidelines for the treatment of neuropathic pain are currently available as discussed and reviewed in Chapter 32 (2, 3). Over the course of his illness, the patient received several first-line drugs for his condition including amitriptyline, gabapentin, pregabalin, and opioids when required. Combining drugs with different mechanisms of action is a long-standing practice in the clinical setting. Randomized controlled trials have only recently investigated combination therapies involving gabapentin and morphine (4), oxycodone (5), or nortriptyline (6), or pregabalin and oxycodone (7). The evidence that combination therapy may be more efficient and induce fewer side-effects than higher doses of a single drug is inconclusive. Monotherapy should be attempted first.

Muscle cramps are involuntary, generally painful contractions of a muscle or muscle group. There is a high frequency of occasional muscle cramps in the general population. In many cases, these muscle cramps are idiopathic or induced by exercise or transient electrolyte disturbances. Several neuromuscular disorders, including peripheral neuropathies, neuromyotonia, and metabolic myopathies, lead to episodes of muscle cramp. The best evidence for treatment efficacy is available for quinine, which is associated with uncommon, but serious side-effects such as pancytopenia, cardiac arrhythmia, or visual loss [and has been withdrawn in the USA by the FDA] (8). There is equivocal evidence from class II studies that magnesium may be helpful. Other class II studies involving diltiazem hydrochloride, naftidrofuryl, and vitamin B complex confirmed some degree of effectiveness. There are no data from clinical trials for frequently used drugs such as baclofen, carbamazepine, and oxcarbazepine.

Our patient with vasculitic neuropathy was prone to adverse drug effects, experiencing several in a predictable manner. Corticosteroids led to severe osteoporosis and an osteoporotic fracture despite regular prophylaxis. Azathioprine was prescribed on several occasions by different physicians, and gastrointestinal side-effects occurred each time. The sodium channel antiepileptics carbamazepine and oxcarbazepine, which efficiently reduced his muscle cramps, also induced severe hyponatremia. The attempt to change from an oral slow-release opioid to transdermal fentanyl led to opioid intoxication. Phenytoin, which also reduced the cramps and was well tolerated, led to intoxication when an intercurrent infection occurred. Fortunately, all of these adverse effects were reversible. A further striking aspect was the marked improvement in both pain and gait when the previously grieving widower developed a relationship with a new companion.

Given the asymmetric onset of a sensorimotor neuropathy with pronounced pain, the suggestive morphology in the sural nerve and some signs of an inflammatory constellation (xANCA positive, oligoclonal bands in the CSF), a diagnosis of NSVN was made in this patient. There are no randomized controlled trials involving drug therapy for NSVN (9). Corticosteroid monotherapy for at least 6 months is considered first-line (10). Combination therapy is considered necessary for rapidly progressive NSVN and patients who have success with corticosteroid monotherapy. Once remission is induced, cyclophosphamide should be replaced with azathioprine or methotrexate. Although the long-term outcome is reasonably positive for most patients, more than one third relapse and a few may die from the disease or treatment complications (11).

Pain in vasculitic neuropathy

Eighty to ninety percent of patients with vasculitic neuropathy experience pain (12). The pain itself is not different from that in other peripheral neuropathies except that it can be focally or multifocally accentuated. Although the multiplex distribution is considered typical for vasculitic neuropathy however, the neuropathy (and consequently the pain) has a distal symmetric distribution in approximately 70% of patients. Immunosuppressive treatment may alleviate pain in some patients. However, a study that examined a large cohort of patients reported that 41% still experienced pain after combination therapy (12).

Vasculitic neuropathy is a classic example of pain induced by a combination of nerve injury and inflammation. The nerve fibers suffer axonal damage through the vasculitis, either by direct ischemic injury or through inflammatory injury. C-fibers are involved in most cases (11). Pro-inflammatory cytokines, which are strong mediators of pain (13), are increased in sural nerve biopsies of vasculitic neuropathy (14). Furthermore, patients with painful neuropathy have higher systemic levels of pro-inflammatory cytokines (15). Combining anti-inflammatory with anti-neuropathic treatment may be an effective strategy for pain control in vasculitic neuropathy although this has not been formally investigated.

References

(1) Treede RD, Jensen TS, Campbell JN, et al. Neuropathic pain: redefinition and a grading system for clinical and research purposes. *Neurology* 2008;70:1630–1635.

(2) Dworkin RH, O'Connor AB, Audette J, et al. Recommendations for the pharmacological management of neuropathic pain: an overview and literature update. *Mayo Clin Proc* 2010;85:S3–S14.

(3) Attal N, Cruccu G, Baron R, et al. EFNS guidelines on the pharmacological treatment of neuropathic pain: 2010 revision. *Eur J Neurol* 2010;17:1113-e88.

(4) Gilron I, Bailey JM, Tu D, Holden RR, Weaver DF, Houlden RL. Morphine, gabapentin, or their combination for neuropathic pain. *N Engl J Med* 2005;352:1324–1334.

(5) Hanna M, O'Brien C, Wilson MC. Prolonged-release oxycodone enhances the effects of existing gabapentin therapy in painful diabetic neuropathy patients. *Eur J Pain* 2008;12:804–813.

(6) Gilron I, Bailey JM, Tu D, Holden RR, Jackson AC, Houlden RL. Nortriptyline and gabapentin, alone and in combination for neuropathic pain: a double-blind, randomised controlled crossover trial. *Lancet* 2009;374:1252–1261.

(7) Gatti A, Sabato AF, Occhioni R, Colini Baldeschi G, Reale C. Controlled-release oxycodone and pregabalin in the treatment of neuropathic pain: results of a multicenter Italian study. *Eur Neurol* 2009;61:129–137.

(8) Katzberg HD, Khan AH, So YT. Assessment: symptomatic treatment for muscle cramps (an evidence-based review): report of the therapeutics and technology assessment subcommittee of the American Academy of Neurology. *Neurology* 2010;74:691–696.

(9) Vrancken AF, Hughes RA, Said G, Wokke JH, Notermans NC. Immunosuppressive treatment for non-systemic vasculitic neuropathy. *Cochrane Database Syst Rev* 2007:CD006050.

(10) Collins MP, Dyck PJB, Gronseth GS, et al. Peripheral Nerve Society Guideline on the classification, diagnosis, investigation, and immunosuppressive therapy of nonsystemic vasculitic neuropathy: executive summary. *J Peripher Nerv Syst* 2010;15:176–184.

(11) Collins MP, Periquet-Collins I. Nonsystemic vasculitic neuropathy: update on diagnosis, classification, pathogenesis, and treatment. *Front Neurol Neurosci* 2009;26:26–66.

(12) Collins MP, Periquet MI, Mendell JR, Sahenk Z, Nagaraja HN, Kissel JT. Nonsystemic vasculitic neuropathy: insights from a clinical cohort. *Neurology* 2003;61:623–630.

(13) Üçeyler N, Schäfers M, Sommer C. Mode of action of cytokines on nociceptive neurons. *Exp Brain Res* 2009;196:67–78.

(14) Lindenlaub T, Sommer C. Cytokines in sural nerve biopsies from inflammatory and non-inflammatory neuropathies. *Acta Neuropathol* 2003;105:593–602.

(15) Üçeyler N, Rogausch JP, Toyka KV, Sommer C. Differential expression of cytokines in painful and painless neuropathies. *Neurology* 2007;69:42–49.

Chapter

13

Painful polyneuropathy associated with anti-MAG autoantibodies

Neuropathic pain may be the presenting feature in patients with polyneuropathy, and may progress in tandem with the disease. While painful polyneuropathies are often erroneously classified as "small fiber" in type, several types may actually be associated with intractable pain. We discuss pain in a patient with an autoimmune, sensory predominant polyneuropathy, particularly involving "large fibers" and originating as an autoimmune attack against myelin, not axons.

Clinical case vignette

A 67-year-old right-handed female retired medical secretary presented with a 1-year history of sensory alteration in the left foot that began in the left large toe. The symptoms progressed to the right foot 2 months later. The patient described the sensation as "something under my feet" with an insensitivity to cold. She experienced "prickling" as well and her walking balance declined. She denied specific weakness of muscles, sphincter dysfunction, or symptoms in her upper limbs. The patient had a history of mild type 2 diabetes mellitus, pernicious anemia, hypercholesterolemia, and ulcerative colitis. There was no family history of polyneuropathy.

Neurological examination disclosed intact mental function, cranial nerves, motor power, muscle bulk, and upper limb coordination. Ankle reflexes were absent but other deep tendon reflexes were intact. There was partial loss of sensation to light touch, pinprick, and temperature in the distal foot and there was complete loss of vibration perception in her large toes. Sensory examination in the upper limbs was normal. Position testing of the toes was also normal. She was mildly unsteady on her feet, but there was no Romberg sign.

Electrophysiological studies identified several abnormalities. The distal motor latencies of the median, ulnar, peroneal, and tibial nerves were prolonged [Figure 13.1]. There was diffuse slowing

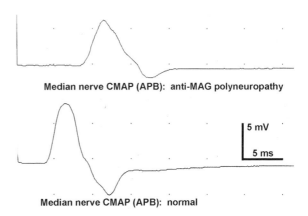

Median nerve CMAP (APB): anti-MAG polyneuropathy

5 mV

5 ms

Median nerve CMAP (APB): normal

Figure 13.1. Electrophysiological studies from the patient described in this vignette. The tracings are CMAPs recorded from the abductor pollicus brevis on stimulation at the wrist. The top tracing is from the patient and the lower tracing from a control subject. Note the prolonged distal motor latency and dispersed appearance of the CMAP from the patient. Patients with anti-MAG polyneuropathy have pronounced demyelination in distal segments, as illustrated.

of motor conduction velocities (e.g., ulnar 30 m/s, N > 50 m/s; peroneal 35 m/s; N > 39 m/s), mild reductions in the amplitudes of the CMAPs, and temporal dispersion of CMAPs with more proximal stimulation. Median and ulnar sensory nerve action potentials (SNAPs) were absent and the sural potentials were reduced in amplitude with mild conduction velocity slowing (2.4 µV, 36 m/s; N > 6 µV, > 39 m/s). Needle electrode examination of the tibialis anterior and extensor digitorum brevis was normal. Overall, the studies identified a widespread sensorimotor polyneuropathy with features of primary demyelination.

Serum protein electrophoresis identified a monoclonal gammopathy (1.3 g/L) characterized as IgMκ. Bone marrow and lymph node biopsies and skeletal survey were normal. Other blood work including complete blood count, sedimentation rate, fasting glucose, CK, ALT, cholesterol, triglycerides, HDL, LDL, B12

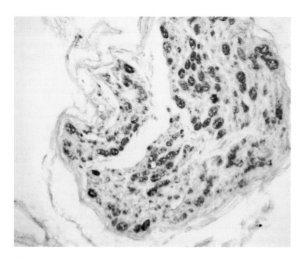

Figure 13.2. Transverse section of a sural nerve immunoreacted with serum from a separate patient with anti-MAG polyneuropathy. Note the selective immunoreactivity of the myelin sheaths indicating immunoreactivity of IgM antibodies in this serum with a myelin antigen. Bar = 20 μm.

level, folate, TSH, and autoantibodies to Yo, Hu, and SS-A/Ro were normal. ANA was positive at 1:160 but anti-DNA was negative. IgM to MAG (myelin-associated glycoprotein) at a titer of 80,000 (Washington University, St. Louis; N < 1500) was positive. A right sural nerve biopsy identified loss of axons, myelin thinning, occasional endoneurial lymphocytes, and on teased analysis, both segmental and paranodal demyelination. Immunohistochemistry demonstrated IgM localized to the myelin sheaths (illustrated in a separate patient in Figure 13.2).

The patient noted increased numbness and more prominent discomfort over the next 2 years. Examination identified a gradual progression in her sensory loss. IVIG therapy was initiated and was associated with a subjective improvement in balance, discomfort, and sensory loss. Despite regular monthly IVIG treatments over the next 5 years, however, there was overall clinical and electrophysiological evidence of gradual deterioration of her polyneuropathy. Sensory loss progressed to the thigh level and involved the hands and distal forearms. She developed mild toe extension weakness and suffered several falls because of a decline in her balance. Her neuropathic pain became more prominent.

Pain description

The patient described several types of discomfort including a sensation that her feet were uncomfort-

ably cold, encased in concrete or that "someone was pulling" her toes upward. She felt cramping in her foot muscles and red hot itchy sensations in her hands. Her most prominent symptom was uncomfortable paresthesiae (tingling) in her feet throughout the day and night. She ranked the pain as 5–6/10 during the day and 10/10 at night. Aching, burning, and electrical-like shocks were additional descriptors. Her pain was associated with frustration, anger, and loneliness and contributed to her balance difficulties. She experienced some benefit from gabapentin but was reluctant to use more than 300 mg at night because of cognitive side-effects.

Discussion

This patient developed an autoimmune peripheral neuropathy associated with antibodies directed against myelin-associated glycoprotein (MAG), a constituent of normal myelin. Her progressive sensory loss, loss of balance, and uncomfortable positive sensory symptoms were classic features of this condition. In addition, her descriptors of paresthesiae (tingling), burning, and electrical-like sensations confirmed the diagnosis of neuropathic pain. Anti-MAG polyneuropathy is particularly directed toward myelin in large axons and the patient's electrophysiological features identified prominent demyelination, especially in very distal nerves (prolonged distal motor latencies). Her biopsy confirmed demyelination but also identified loss of axons, an additional feature of the disease. Although she had mild type 2 diabetes mellitus, she was not thought to have superimposed diabetic neuropathy. Although IVIG and gabapentin provided some relief, their effects were incomplete and significantly interfered with her quality of life. Such incomplete responses typically decrease patient interest to currently available forms of therapy. Otherwise high functioning individuals often prefer not to use opioids or other agents because of their cognitive side-effects.

Pain in anti-MAG polyneuropathy

Because multiple mechanisms can potentially generate neuropathic pain, understanding how it arises in an individual patient may be difficult. First, it seems difficult to reconcile prominent pain in a patient in whom an autoimmune attack is directed at myelin, and not the axon itself. Neuropathic pain however, is common in demyelinating polyneuropathies including Guillain-Barré syndrome (1) and chronic inflammatory demyelinating polyneuropathy (CIDP) (2). In the two patients described in (2), severe and deep boring upper limb pain predicted early relapses of CIDP that eventually required further therapy (2). It may be that the inflammatory response associated with demyelinating neuropathies triggers ectopic discharges of nearby "bystander" axons: mediators might include TNFα, nitric oxide, bradykinin, interleukins, or others (3–6). The critical role of Schwann cells, the chief supporting cells of the peripheral nervous system for axons and neurons, must also be considered. Without such support, axons may become dysfunctional and degenerate, a process in itself that might trigger ectopic painful discharges through abnormal sodium channel distributions or kinetics. Alterations in the peptide content of the parent axon or cell body in the sensory ganglion is an additional source of painful ectopic discharges in neuropathic pain (7, 8). In our patient, lymphocytes capable of releasing inflammatory mediators had indeed entered the nerve and axons had also been destroyed. Finally, some have postulated that internodes denuded of myelin are capable of generating ectopic activity through recruitment of neighbor axons, or ephactic transmission (9).

Initial treatment for neuropathic pain from polyneuropathy probably should begin with better tolerated agents such as gabapentin, other antiepileptics, followed by tricyclic antidepressants (such as amitriptyline) and finally opioids. Evidence-based guidelines for the priority in initiating these agents has been debated and consensus statements are summarized in Chapter 32. Low-dose opioid therapy (oxycontin, fentanyl patches, slow-release morphine) can be a safe and effective approach in patients with significant cardiac or renal comorbidity but constipation and cognitive side-effects are frequent.

References

(1) Moulin DE, Hagen N, Feasby TE, Amireh R, Hahn A. Pain in Guillain-Barré syndrome. *Neurology* 1997;48: 328–331.

(2) Zochodne DW, Brunet DG. Upper limb pain in chronic demyelinating polyneuropathy: electrophysiological correlates. *Acta Neurol Scand* 1994;90:270–275.

(3) Sommer C, Lindenlaub T, Teuteberg P, Schafers M, Hartung T, Toyka KV. Anti-TNF-neutralizing antibodies reduce pain-related behavior in two different mouse models of painful mononeuropathy. *Brain Res* 2001;913:86–89.

(4) Levy D, Zochodne DW. Local nitric oxide synthase activity in a model of neuropathic pain. *Eur J Neurosci* 1998;10:1846–1855.

(5) Levy D, Zochodne DW. Increased mRNA expression of the B1 and B2 bradykinin receptors and antinociceptive effects of their antagonists in an animal model of neuropathic pain. *Pain* 2000;86: 265–271.

(6) Rowbotham MC, Petersen KL, Davies PS, Friedman EK, Fields HL. Recent developments in the treatment of neuropathic pain. In: Devor M, Rowbotham MC, Wiesenfeld-Hallin Z, eds. *Proceedings of the 9th World Congress of Pain*. Seattle: IASP Press, 2000: 833–855.

(7) Cummins TR, Dib-Hajj S, Black JA, Waxman SG. Sodium channels as molecular targets in pain. In: Devor M, Rowbotham MC, Wiesenfeld-Hallin Z, eds. *Proceedings of the 9th World Congress on Pain*. Seattle: IASP Press, 2000:77–91.

(8) Devor M. The pathophysiology of damaged peripheral nerves. In: Wall PD, Melzack R, eds. *Textbook of Pain*. 4th edition. London: Churchill Livingston, 1994:79–100.

(9) Amir R, Devor M. Axonal cross-excitation in nerve-end neuromas: comparison of A- and C-fibers. *J Neurophysiol* 1992;68:1160–1166.

Painful polyneuropathy associated with inherited amyloidosis

The polyneuropathy associated with amyloidosis classically involves small caliber sensory and autonomic axons early, and is often associated with prominent neuropathic pain. This chapter describes a patient with late-onset inherited amyloidosis-related polyneuropathy.

Clinical case vignette

This 72-year-old right-handed male of Danish extraction developed symptoms approximately 5 years before evaluation. He described "cold" feet that evolved into painful, burning sensations in a stocking distribution also associated with paresthesiae. The symptoms gradually progressed proximally up his legs and involved his finger tips 2 years before presentation. Six months before his visit, he noticed a decline in balance with falls in the shower, clumsiness in his fine finger movements, and allodynia. Other symptoms included a decline in grip strength, difficulty arising from chairs, and erectile dysfunction. Bowel and bladder dysfunction or postural lightheadedness were denied although diarrhea had developed just before the visit.

A prior lumbar laminectomy, cholecystectomy, and borderline diabetes mellitus were reported. There was no definite history of polyneuropathy involving his parents, a sister, or three sons, although his father died at a young age for unrelated reasons.

On neurological examination, mental status, speech, and cranial nerves were intact. He had wasting of his intrinsic hand muscles and lower limb pitting edema. There was weakness of his hand muscles (4/5) and in foot dorsiflexion, plantar flexion, inversion, and eversion (3/5). Lower limb reflexes were absent, and there was loss of sensation distal to the knees and proximal fingers. There was loss of sensitivity to light touch distal to his knees and analgesia and anesthesia in his toes. He had loss of vibration sensation in his toes, made errors with position sensation testing, and

walked with an unsteady steppage gait. An inability to stand on his toes or his heels accompanied a Romberg sign. There was no significant postural blood pressure drop with standing.

Electrophysiological studies identified widespread severe reductions or loss of CMAP amplitudes. Distal motor latencies were prolonged in the median and ulnar nerves at the wrists and there was slowing of forearm ulnar motor and leg peroneal motor conduction velocity. SNAPs were markedly reduced in amplitude with patchy slowing of conduction velocities in the upper limbs. SNAPs were absent in the lower limbs. Needle electrode study of tibialis anterior and vastus lateralis identified fibrillation potentials, positive sharp waves, and a reduced number of enlarged motor unit potentials with an increased firing rate.

Normal (negative) laboratory studies included: complete blood count, ESR, INR, electrolytes, fasting glucose, calcium, magnesium, urinalysis, venous lactate, alkaline phosphatase, ALT, AST, bilirubin (total and direct), ferritin, GGT, LDH, total protein, albumin, B12, TSH, HbA1C, lipid profile, cryoglobulin, serum protein electrophoresis, urine protein electrophoresis, immunofixation, quantitative immunoglobulins, antibodies to sulfatide and MAG, RF, and skeletal survey. A CK level was mildly elevated at 263 U/L (normal, <195). The ANA screen was positive at 1:320 and showed a nucleolar pattern. Bone density scores in the spine and femoral neck were in the osteoporotic range. A CT scan of the chest (and plain chest film) and abdomen identified atelectasis in the left costophrenic angle and right middle lobe and hypertrophy of the left ventricle, but the studies were otherwise normal. An electrocardiogram showed normal sinus rhythm, nonspecific T wave abnormalities inferolaterally and low voltage QRS limb leads. A two-dimensional echocardiogram identified increased thickness of the right and left ventricles with normal function, biatrial enlargement, and mild mitral and tricuspid regurgitation.

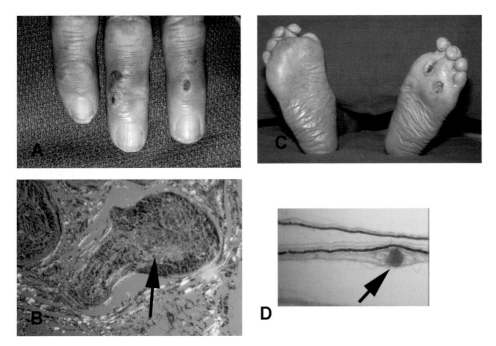

Figure 14.1 Images illustrating amyloid polyneuropathy in patients other than described in the clinical vignette. Images A and B show examples of self-injury and ulceration in the finger tips and feet of a patient who had amputations of his large toes because of ulceration and infection. This patient had acquired amyloidosis with severe amyloid polyneuropathy and insensitivity to injury. Images C and D illustrate histological examples of amyloid deposition in a transverse section of a sural nerve illuminated by polarized light and stained with Congo red. The arrow points to apple-green birefringence surrounding an endoneurial vessel. In D, illustrated is a teased myelinated axon with a large amyloid deposit (arrow) adjacent to and partly compressing it.

A right sural nerve biopsy showed severe loss of myelinated axons, hyalinized endoneurial and perineurial blood vessels that were birefringent green on Congo red staining with polarized light, rare macrophages without an inflammatory infiltrate, and other endoneurial amyloid deposits. The findings identified a severe neuropathy with evidence of amyloidosis. Amyloidosis was confirmed and was linked to a V30M mutation of the TTR (transthyretin) gene [courtesy of Amyloid Treatment and Research Program, Boston Medical University, Dr. Martha Skinner].

Two years following his visit, the patient required admission to hospital with urinary retention, pneumonia, weight loss, and right-sided cardiac failure. He died 3 months later at home.

Pain description

During 2 years of follow-up, this patient's primary difficulty was his severe and intractable neuropathic pain that routinely interrupted his sleep. He described burning hyperalgesia, paresthesiae, allody-nia, and spasms. It was aggravated by walking, long standing, or sitting. Partial relief was achieved with gabapentin, amitriptyline, and oxycontin. High doses of gabapentin were associated with diarrhea, whereas opioids induced severe constipation and nausea. He described progressive daily pain extending from his feet to his hips.

Discussion

This patient had a severe and progressive sensory and motor polyneuropathy associated with familial amyloidotic polyneuropathy (FAP). Amyloidosis refers to a spectrum of systemic and neurological disorders associated with the deposition of protein that exhibits apple-green birefringent fluorescence under a fluorescence microscope when the tissue is stained with Congo red dye (see review (1))[Figure 14.1C,D]. Amyloidosis involving the peripheral nervous system can be primary acquired, associated with deposits of immunoglobulin light chains, or familial as described in this case. Familial amyloidosis was originally classified as FAP Types I–IV, but is currently associated with transthyretin mutations (Type I, Portuguese or Andrade; Type II Indiana-Swiss, or Rukavina), apolipoprotein A-I mutations (Type III Iowa or Van Allen), and gelsolin mutations (Type IV Finnish or Meretoja).

V30M (valine is substituted with methionine), the mutation in our patient, is the most common of the transthyretin mutations, is autosomal dominant and linked to FAP Type I and II. This was also the mutation discovered in the original Portuguese or Andrade kindred. While V30M transthyretin amyloidosis was originally described as FAPI and identified in patients from Portugal, Japan, Sweden, and the USA, it is 1 of over 100 mutations identified in the primary structure of transthyretin, a plasma transport protein for thyroid hormone and retinol-binding protein (2). The onset has been described as late in Sweden, as in our patient, but early in Portugal. V30M is associated with peripheral neuropathy, carpal tunnel syndrome, autonomic neuropathy, and vitreous opacities. Painful burning feet may be an initial symptom of peripheral neuropathy. Loss of small fiber sensory modalities is prominent (pain and temperature sensation) in a stocking and glove distribution. Self-injury and ulceration may develop from loss of protective sensation [Figure 14.1A,B]. Distal lower limb weakness is common and autonomic symptoms include postural lightheadedness from postural hypotension, bowel and bladder emptying abnormalities, impotence, and sweating loss (1). Electrophysiological studies show evidence of a progressive axonal sensory and motor polyneuropathy, as observed in our patient, with superimposed carpal tunnel syndrome. Ocular abnormalities include scalloped pupils, vitreous opacities mentioned above, keratoconjunctivitis sicca, and glaucoma. It remains unclear how the variant protein generates axonal damage in FAP, but it is thought to be neurotoxic. Despite his late onset, our patient had no clear family history of the condition, normally displayed in an autosomal dominant inheritance pattern. Some instances are secondary to spontaneous de novo mutations and penetrance may be as low as 50%.

The clinical, electrophysiological and biopsy results of probands from 35 families in Japan with V30M FAP were reviewed by Misu et al. (3). While neuropathic pain was not specifically mentioned in this group, initial paresthesiae were the most common initial complaint. The patients were late-onset (from age 50), predominantly male, and had a family history in only one third of instances. Few autonomic symptoms were reported. At autopsy in three patients, amyloid deposits were noted in the sympathetic ganglia, dorsal root ganglia, and peripheral nerve trunks, and were associated with axonal degeneration. Unmyelinated axons were relatively spared, a possible reason for the prominent symptoms of pain described in other series of patients with late onset V30M FAP. Overall the changes were thought less severe than those of early onset amyloidosis. Autonomic difficulties included postural hypotension, occasional syncope, alternating diarrhea and constipation, urinary retention, male sexual impotence, and distal loss of sweating. Patients most often had panmodal loss of sensation, greater lower limb than upper limb weakness and in the heart, cardiac conduction abnormalities or hypertrophy.

Our patient's disease course was relentless and progressive with evidence of gastrointestinal (diarrhea alternating with constipation) and cardiac (ventricular wall thickening and later right heart failure) involvement. Beyond orthotopic liver transplantation, not considered for our patient because of his advanced age, effective treatment for FAP is limited.

Pain in amyloid-associated polyneuropathy

While the prevalence of pain in FAP patients is thought to be high, exact figures are difficult to ascertain. In a series of ten patients selected for liver transplantation in Boston, five had lancinating pain that improved after the transplant (4). It is uncertain whether deposits of amyloid proteins in nerve trunks or ganglia might signal specific pain receptors or channels. Painful amyloid polyneuropathy has been identified as an example of "small fiber" neuropathy. Why loss of small fibers should generate pain rather than analgesia is problematic. Targeting of small axons and their ganglia perikarya before frank drop out may be a reasonable explanation for this clinical syndrome. While polyneuropathy in amyloidosis is often associated with selective small axon loss, our patient's nerve biopsy identified widespread loss of both myelinated and unmyelinated axons in addition to amyloid deposition. His pain descriptors indicated neuropathic pain with burning, uncomfortable paresthesiae and allodynia. The difficulties of current pharmacological therapy for severe neuropathic pain were illustrated by the patient's severe gastrointestinal side-effects that ensued in attempting to titrate his analgesics.

Despite the use of higher doses, his symptoms were only partially relieved.

References

(1) Mendell JR. Familial amyloid polyneuropathies. In: Mendell JR, Kissel JT, Cornblath DR, eds. *Diagnosis and Management of Peripheral Nerve Disorders*. Oxford: Oxford University Press, 2001:477–491.

(2) Benson MD, Kincaid JC. The molecular biology and clinical features of amyloid neuropathy. *Muscle Nerve* 2007;36:411–423.

(3) Misu K, Hattori N, Nagamatsu M, et al. Late-onset familial amyloid polyneuropathy type I (transthyretin Met30-associated familial amyloid polyneuropathy) unrelated to endemic focus in Japan. Clinicopathological and genetic features. *Brain* 1999;122(Pt 10): 1951–1962.

(4) Pomfret EA, Lewis WD, Jenkins RL, et al. Effect of orthotopic liver transplantation on the progression of familial amyloidotic polyneuropathy. *Transplantation* 1998;65:918–925.

Chapter

15

Small fiber neuropathy in sarcoidosis

This patient vignette illustrates how a neuropathic pain syndrome may lead to an unexpected underlying diagnosis. Unexplained pain in sarcoidosis may guide the way toward a diagnosis of small fiber neuropathy.

Clinical case vignette

A 50-year-old female physician presented with burning pain in the soles of her feet and the palms of her hands. She had been taking nonsteroidal anti-inflammatory drugs without effect. Her medical history was unremarkable except for arterial hypertension and obesity. Neurological examination was normal. Nerve conduction studies gave normal results in the motor nerves and showed moderate reduction of sensory nerve action potential amplitudes in the left sural nerve. The sympathetic skin response in the arms and legs was normal. Quantitative sensory testing revealed a moderately increased detection threshold for warm temperatures in the feet, with normal thresholds for all other sensory qualities, and normal thresholds in the hands. Laboratory investigations including serum chemistry, complete blood count, erythrocyte sedimentation rate, serum vitamin B12 concentration, serum protein electrophoresis, antinuclear antibodies, and angiotensin-converting enzyme (ACE) were all normal. Cerebrospinal fluid, including the ACE level, was also normal.

An initial and tentative diagnosis of small fiber neuropathy (SFN) was made; a skin punch biopsy was performed and processed for analysis of skin innervation and inflammatory cells. In a sample taken from the lower leg, intraepidermal nerve fiber density (IENFD) was reduced to 3.3 fibers/mm (normal, 9.5 ± 3), and IENFD from the upper thigh, at 9 fibers/mm, was in the lower range of normal. The results confirmed a length-dependent small fiber neuropathy [Figure 15.1A,B]. Dermal macrophages and T-lymphocytes were also moderately increased [Figure 15.1C,D].

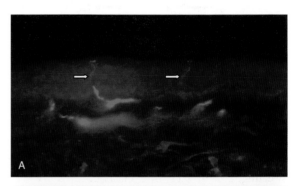

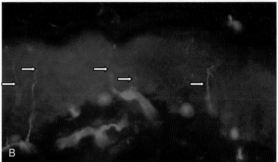

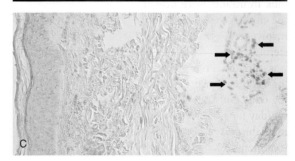

Figure 15.1 Skin biopsy from the lower (A) and upper (B) leg of the patient. (A, B) Immunofluorescent staining with antibodies to PGP 9.5 to visualize intra- and subepidermal nerve fibers (arrows). Note reduction of nerve fibers in (A). (C) Immunohistochemical stains for macrophages and T lymphocytes (arrows) in the subepidermal skin. The presence of granulomas is notably absent.

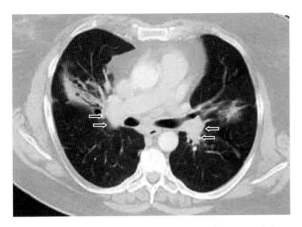

Figure 15.2 Computerized tomography scan of the patient's lung showing bihilar mediastinal lymph node enlargement (arrows). Images: courtesy of Prof. Hahn, Inst. for Radiology, University Hospital of Würzburg.

Because the patient also complained of weight loss of 4 kg in the last 3 months as well as increased sweating, a chest x-ray and subsequently a CT scan of the thorax were done; bihilar mediastinal lymph node enlargement was found [Figure 15.2]. Pulmonary function testing showed a moderate restrictive ventilatory impairment. Lymphoma and sarcoidosis were considered as differential diagnoses. Bronchial lavage revealed 15% of lymphocytic cells in flow cytometry, mostly T-lymphocytes, with an increased CD4/CD8 ratio of 3.3 (normal: 1.1–2.5). Transbronchial biopsy of the lymph nodes revealed non-caseating epithelioid granulomas, typical of sarcoidosis. Granulomatous infiltrates were also found in a skin biopsy of the chin. A diagnosis of sarcoidosis with multi-organ involvement was made and treatment with corticosteroids, complemented by osteoporosis prophylaxis, was initiated. Prednisolone was initiated at a dose of 1 mg/kg, then slowly tapered to a maintenance dose of 20 mg daily and later supplemented by azathioprine 150 mg/day for steroid sparing. Under this treatment regimen, the pain was markedly reduced and symptomatic treatment for neuropathic pain was not required. Approximately 6 months after the diagnosis had been made, the prednisolone dose was reduced to 10 mg, and shortly after that, pain resumed. A complete internal medical and neurological check-up revealed no major changes, except that sural nerve conduction studies were now normal. The prednisolone dose was increased to 15 mg daily for several weeks and later again reduced to 10 mg. When the patient was seen again 1 year later, she was generally improved, pul-

monary function was almost normalized, the mediastinal lymph nodes had become smaller, and the patient did not complain of pain. Prednisolone was further tapered. One year later, now under 6 mg daily of prednisolone, the patient reported intermittent increases of the burning acral pain, which spontaneously resolved after several days. She did not wish symptomatic treatment for neuropathic pain.

Pain description

In the initial phase of her disease, the patient described burning pain and a tingling in the soles of her feet while at rest as well as in the palms of her hands. She ranked her pain at 4–5/10 when at rest. When touched by clothing or after prolonged standing, her pain severity could increase to 8/10. After the initiation of treatment, the pain was markedly reduced, but the patient noticed a sensation of numbness in the areas that had previously been painful.

Discussion

Sarcoidosis is a disseminated granulomatous disease of presumed auto-immune origin. There may be a genetic disposition (1, 2). Exogenous causative factors ranging from drugs to pollen and viruses are also suspect. The *Mycobacterium tuberculosis* catalase-peroxidase (mKatG) protein is a potential antigen (3). The prevalence of sarcoidosis ranges from 1–40 per 100,000 among various ethnic and racial groups. Almost all organs may be impacted, most often lung, liver, skin, and eyes. The disease is chronic and progressive in approximately 25% of cases. Neurosarcoidosis with CNS involvement has been estimated at 10% of all cases (4), but this statistic may be underestimated (5). Neurosarcoidosis mimics most CNS diseases and consequently, a list of differential diagnoses can be long (6). Treatment options include corticosteroids, azathioprine and methotrexate. Anti-tumor necrosis factor-alpha (TNF) therapy has also been used (7).

Sarcoid peripheral neuropathy has long been recognized, often described as a vasculitis-like neuropathy with typical granulomas in the nerve (8– 10). In a Dutch treatment center for this disease, almost 50% of all patients complained of pain and paresthesias in the distal extremities (11). The suspicion that these patients might be suffering from small fiber neuropathy (SFN) was subsequently confirmed by QST and by quantification of skin innervation. Many patients also had symptoms of autonomic dysfunction. Other

67

potential causes of SFN were excluded. Sarcoidosis therapy, such as corticosteroids or TNF inhibitors, may help alleviate SFN symptoms (12). Patients responsive to intravenous immunoglobulins have also been described (13). When sufficient immunosuppressive treatment of sarcoidosis is given and pain persists, medications for neuropathic pain may be prescribed (14); data for the most effective treatment regimen are unavailable (14).

Small fiber neuropathies are a subtype of sensory neuropathies exclusively or predominately affecting small diameter nerve fibers, and are discussed in more detail in Chapter 11. These include small diameter myelinated fibers (A∂) and unmyelinated (C) fibers. Both sensory and autonomic fibers may be involved. The typical and most common presentation is a complaint of burning feet (15). In the patient described above, SFN was the first manifestation of sarcoidosis. The history of weight loss and increased sweating triggered a more extensive diagnostic workup, including chest x-ray, which eventually led to the diagnosis.

Pain in sarcoidosis

Patients with sarcoidosis experience several types of pain; the SFN-related pain represents one of several. In a Dutch survey of over 800 patients, 72% complained of pain. Arthralgia was the most frequent (53.8%), followed by muscle pain (40.2%), headache (28.0%), and chest pain (26.9%). Patients with more types of pain had impaired indices of their quality of life. The typical and most common presentation of SFN is a complaint of burning feet. Approximately 50% of patients have paresthesias, lancinating pain, and negative symptoms including numbness (15, 16). The initial presentation is in the feet; the hands may become involved over time. The persistent pain is variously described as burning, prickling, or deep and aching. Lancinating pains are described as brief, stabbing, or like electric shocks. The feet may feel cold, or feel as if the skin is too tight. Patients may also complain of thermal hypersensitivity. Pain is often worse at rest, particularly at night, and may interfere with sleep. Allodynia may make bedsheets intolerable and prevent patients from wearing certain footwear.

The mere loss of skin innervation is not necessarily associated with pain (17). For example, patients with motor neuron disease and no pain may have considerable loss of small fibers in the skin (18). In these instances, additional factors in the damaged

nerve fibers or in their environment may be responsible for inducing sensations of pain. Because small fiber neuropathy is characterized by localized pain, local increases in inflammatory mediators, which then activate and sensitize nociceptors, may play a role. Dysregulated cytokine inflammatory mediators in the skin may be a factor explaining pain in sarcoidosis (1). In idiopathic length-dependent SFN, local skin cytokine profiles are shifted to a proinflammatory status within involved body areas (19). In the subgroup of patients with small fiber neuropathy, cytokine expression in the painful skin was greatly increased compared with uninvolved skin. Thus, local increases in pro-inflammatory cytokines like TNF may be involved in the pathophysiology of pain in small fiber neuropathy. Whether this is true in sarcoid SFN, or whether other inflammatory mediators are more important in this disorder, requires clarification.

Treatment in sarcoidosis is dependent on the extent of organ involvement. Most patients with sarcoidosis require no specific treatment (1). When treatment is necessary, patients usually improve with moderate doses of corticosteroids. However, long-standing corticosteroid treatment leads to unwanted side-effects. TNF inhibitors have been investigated for the treatment of sarcoidosis, but are not yet recommended for use. Immunosuppressants including azathioprine, methotrexate, cyclosporine, and cyclophosphamide are used, particularly in cases involving neurosarcoidosis (6), but evidence-based data from trials are unavailable. The pain in sarcoid SFN is frequently alleviated by immunosuppressive treatment. If this is not sufficient, symptomatic treatment may be attempted with medications used for other types of neuropathic pain including amitriptyline, gabapentin, pregabalin, and others (14). One small controlled trial has given some indication that pain in idiopathic small fiber neuropathy may respond to drugs generally given for neuropathic pain (20). Local treatment options like lidocaine or capsaicin patches may potentially be helpful but there are no controlled data yet on their use in either sarcoid-related or idiopathic SFN.

References

(1) Morgenthau AS, Iannuzzi MC. Recent advances in sarcoidosis. *Chest* 2011;139:174–182.

(2) Hofmann S, Fischer A, Till A, et al. A genome-wide association study reveals evidence of association with sarcoidosis at 6p12.1. *Eur Respir J* 2011;38:1127–1135.

(3) Song Z, Marzilli L, Greenlee BM, et al. Mycobacterial catalase-peroxidase is a tissue antigen and target of the adaptive immune response in systemic sarcoidosis. *J Exp Med* 2005;201:755–767.

(4) Terushkin V, Stern BJ, Judson MA, et al. Neurosarcoidosis: presentations and management. *Neurologist* 2010;16:2–15.

(5) Joseph FG, Scolding NJ. Neurosarcoidosis: a study of 30 new cases. *J Neurol Neurosurg Psychiatry* 2009;80: 297–304.

(6) Hoitsma E, Drent M, Sharma OP. A pragmatic approach to diagnosing and treating neurosarcoidosis in the 21st century. *Curr Opin Pulm Med* 2010;16: 472–479.

(7) Baughman RP, Drent M, Kavuru M, et al. Infliximab therapy in patients with chronic sarcoidosis and pulmonary involvement. *Am J Respir Crit Care Med* 2006;174:795–802.

(8) Galassi G, Gibertoni M, Mancini A, et al. Sarcoidosis of the peripheral nerve: clinical, electrophysiological and histological study of two cases. *Eur Neurol* 1984;23:459–465.

(9) Zuniga G, Ropper AH, Frank J. Sarcoid peripheral neuropathy. *Neurology* 1991;41:1558–1561.

(10) Said G, Lacroix C, Plante-Bordeneuve V, et al. Nerve granulomas and vasculitis in sarcoid peripheral neuropathy: a clinicopathological study of 11 patients. *Brain* 2002;125:264–275.

(11) Hoitsma E, Marziniak M, Faber CG, et al. Small fibre neuropathy in sarcoidosis. *Lancet* 2002;359:2085–2086.

(12) Hoitsma E, Faber CG, van Santen-Hoeufft M, De Vries J, Reulen JP, Drent M. Improvement of small fiber neuropathy in a sarcoidosis patient after treatment with infliximab. *Sarcoidosis Vasc Diffuse Lung Dis* 2006;23:73–77.

(13) Parambil JG, Tavee JO, Zhou L, Pearson KS, Culver DA. Efficacy of intravenous immunoglobulin for small fiber neuropathy associated with sarcoidosis. *Respir Med* 2011;105:101–105.

(14) Attal N, Cruccu G, Baron R, et al. EFNS guidelines on the pharmacological treatment of neuropathic pain: 2010 revision. *Eur J Neurol* 2010;17:1113–e88.

(15) Lacomis D. Small-fiber neuropathy. *Muscle Nerve* 2002;26:173–188.

(16) Sommer C, Lauria G. Chapter 41 Painful small-fiber neuropathies. *Handb Clin Neurol* 2006;81:621–633.

(17) Vlckova-Moravcova E, Bednarik J, Belobradkova J, Sommer C. Small-fibre involvement in diabetic patients with neuropathic foot pain. *Diabet Med* 2008;25:692–699.

(18) Weis J, Katona I, Muller-Newen G, et al. Small-fiber neuropathy in patients with ALS. *Neurology* 2011; 76:2024–2029.

(19) Üçeyler N, Kafke W, Riediger N, et al. Elevated proinflammatory cytokine expression in affected skin in small fiber neuropathy. *Neurology* 2010;74:1806–1813.

(20) Ho TW, Backonja M, Ma J, Leibensperger H, Froman S, Polydefkis M. Efficient assessment of neuropathic pain drugs in patients with small fiber sensory neuropathies. *Pain* 2009;141:19–24.

Chapter 16

Pain and small fiber polyneuropathy in Fabry disease

Fabry disease (FD) is an inherited, X-linked lysosomal storage disorder caused by deficiency of the enzyme α-galactosidase A (α-GAL) (1). The disease is characterized by intracellular deposition of glycosphingolipids (mostly globotriaosylceramide, GL-3) that may involve various organs including the central and peripheral nervous systems. Pain is an early symptom that can facilitate recognition of the disease and in turn, prevent major organ failure through adequate and timely treatment.

Clinical case vignette

A 41-year-old man was diagnosed with FD in April 2004 through the process of family screening after confirmation of FD in his brother. A splicing defect of IVS3 + 1 G > A on the GLA-gene and loss of α-GAL activity were discovered. His medical history included a deep femoral vein thrombosis in 1993 and a myocardial infarction in 1996. Typical Fabry-related symptoms included repeated acute hearing loss, periumbilical angioektasia, and heat intolerance with hypohidrosis. The patient also reported pain in his hands and feet triggered by fever. Kidney function, measured by clearance of technetium-99m-labeled diethylenetriamine pentaacetate (99mTc-DTPA), revealed a glomerular filtration rate (GFR) of 140 mL/min per 1.73 m^2 (normal range, 90–150 mL), without evidence of proteinuria. Echocardiography showed a borderline hypertrophy of the left ventricle with a septum wall thickness of 12 mm (normal range, < 12 mm). Enzyme replacement therapy (ERT) was initiated shortly after the diagnosis of FD was confirmed in April 2004.

The first neurological examination of the patient was performed in April 2007. At that time, cardiac and renal status were within the normal range. The patient reported typical Fabry crises in which he had attacks of severe burning pain in his hands and feet induced by exercise, stress, and temperature changes, including

fever. He had suffered many similar episodes during childhood and into adulthood, with some improvement after initiation of symptomatic treatment with phenytoin. The patient further reported that, under ERT, painful episodes occurred less frequently and were less severe. Heat tolerance was likewise improved. Neurological examination was normal except for evidence of carpal tunnel syndrome (CTS) involving the right hand. Electrodiagnostic studies showed reductions in median nerve SNAP amplitude and nerve conduction velocity (NCV) in combination with a prolonged distal motor latency of the right motor median nerve, confirming CTS. Nerve conduction studies of the left median and the right sural nerve were normal as was the sympathetic skin response at the right foot. Quantitative sensory testing (QST) at the right foot revealed increased cold detection threshold (CDT), warm detection threshold (WDT), and thermal sensitivity threshold (limen) (TSL), indicating loss of function of Aδ- and C-fibers (Table 16.1). A skin punch biopsy was taken from the right lower leg 10 cm above the lateral malleolus [Figure 16.1]. Intraepidermal nerve fiber density was reduced to 1.1 fibers/mm (normal, 10±3 fibers/mm), confirming small-fiber neuropathy.

A follow-up examination was done in April 2008. The patient was in a stable clinical condition, renal and cardiac parameters were within normal ranges. He reported less severe pain and fewer pain attacks during the last year; evaluated with the Graded Chronic Pain Scale (GCPS) (2), he also had lower pain scores (total score of the 1–3 items of GCPS) and pain-related disability (total score of the 5–7 items of GCPS) compared with 2007. The grade of pain severity ameliorated from grade III in 2007 to grade I in 2008 (Table 16.1). Nerve conduction of the right median nerve improved following carpal tunnel surgery in June 2007. In QST of the right foot, thermal thresholds were improved when compared with the previous examination [Table 16.1].

Table 16.1. Neurophysiological findings, quantitative sensory testing, and pain rating

	Right sural nerve NCS		Right median nerve NCS						QST			GCPS scores		
			Sensory			Motor								
	SNAP (μV)	NCV (m/s)	SNAP (μV)	NCV (m/s)	DL (ms)	CMAP (mV)	NCV (m/s)	DML (ms)	CDT (°C)	WDT (°C)	TSL (°C)	Pain intensity*	Pain disability†	Grade of pain severity‡
2007	18.4	50.0	18.0	34.5	4.6	9.1	n.d.	5.8	−22	18	32.7	40	3	III
2008	17.8	47.0	24.0	46.0	3.6	11.7	52.0	4.8	−9.1	11	18.4	30	0	I

Scores derived from *items 1–3, †items 5–7, and ‡items 1–7 of the GCPS questionnaire, related to the 4 weeks previous to examination. CDT: cold detection threshold; CMAP: compound muscle action potential; DML: distal motor latency; GCPS: Graded Clinical Pain Scale; GFR: glomerular filtration rate; IENFD: intraepidermal nerve fiber density; NCS: nerve conduction studies; NCV: nerve conduction velocity; n.d.: not done; QST: quantitative sensory testing; SNAP: sensory nerve action potential; TSL: thermal sensory limen (temperature change needed to detect difference). WDT: Warm detection threshold

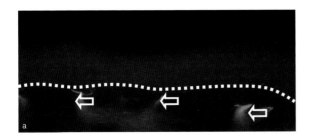

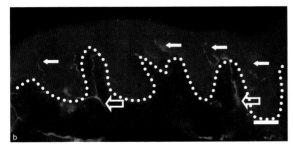

Figure 16.1. (A) Photomicrograph of a section from the patient's skin biopsy from the lower calf. Immunofluorescence with antibodies to the pan-axonal marker protein gene product (PGP) 9.5. Note only subepidermal nerve fibers (open arrows) as compared to that in a section from a control person (B) with numerous intraepidermal nerve fibers (arrows) and subepidermal nerve fibers (open arrows). Bar = 20 μm. Dotted line: Dermal–epidermal junction.

Pain description

Although pain intensity was rated as 4/10 in the weeks preceding the first visit, the patient described intermittent peaks of pain that reached an intensity of 8/10. These peaks were associated with physical exercise, stress, and hot temperatures, including fever. Abrupt temperature changes, no matter in which direction, could also bring on pain crises. The patient characterized the pain as mostly burning although deep aching pain could also occur. In addition, he complained of nightly pain in the right hand which could be attributed to the CTS and was no longer present at the follow-up visit. The patient had learned over the years that standard analgesics were not helpful and that a daily intake of 300 mg phenytoin in divided doses reduced the pain intensity. He took the medication mostly in summer and when he anticipated physical exertion.

Discussion

This patient had experienced typical acral pains related to Fabry disease throughout his life-time. Pain occurred with febrile episodes in his childhood and also with febrile infections in adulthood. Hot ambient temperature and increases of body core temperature through physical exercise also induced pain. Although the patient had further typical Fabry-related symptoms such as hypohidrosis, repeated acute hearing loss, and periumbilical angioektasia, the diagnosis was not made until the patient's more severely affected brother was diagnosed with Fabry's disease. Despite the long duration of disease, the patient was relatively mildly involved; renal function and cardiac function were normal and borderline normal, respectively. In other patients with a similar history, the diagnosis is sometimes made when renal failure has already occurred.

Apart from cardiac and renal involvement, one reason for the limited life expectancy of Fabry patients is central nervous system involvement mainly due to ischemic strokes (3). Along with macroangiopathic changes, Fabry patients frequently develop cerebral microangiopathy that causes progressive white matter lesions (WMLs) (4, 5). This may lead to deterioration of cognitive function.

In the peripheral nervous system, Fabry patients develop a neuropathy primarily involving C-fibers and Aδ-fibers (small-fiber neuropathy) (6–8). Large-fiber involvement is mainly limited to patients in advanced disease stages already suffering from renal impairment. Routine neurophysiological tests selectively evaluate faster conducting myelinated Aα- and Aβ-fibers. To test the function of small nerve fibers, other diagnostic tools are necessary. A bedside test of small-fiber function and quantitative sensory testing (QST) are useful approaches (9–11). Quantitative thermotesting is a psychophysical method of evaluating temperature perception and pain thresholds in various skin areas (9–11). Fabry patients usually show raised thresholds of cold more than warm perception (9, 12, 13). With these findings, and after more common causes of small-fiber neuropathy (such as diabetes mellitus or alcohol abuse) are excluded, the diagnosis of Fabry disease should be considered and an enzyme test performed. It is assumed that small-fiber neuropathy is mainly due to GL-3 deposits in the dorsal root ganglion (DRG) neurons which may also be a cause for the pain. The vulnerability of small DRG neurons in this condition and the triggering of pain to temperature changes is not yet understood.

ERT may reduce neuropathic pain, but larger trials are needed to confirm this (14, 15). Some patients may substantially reduce their pain medication when under ERT. Others find that ERT provokes pain, particularly in the early stages of treatment, and symptomatic treatment is required. Improvement of small fiber function under ERT has been established in previous investigations as assessed by QST (14, 15). In this patient, small fiber function had also considerably improved (Table 16.1) after 1 year of follow-up.

A very common manifestation of Fabry disease is hypohidrosis, which may lead to heat intolerance. Hypohidrosis is presumably the consequence of both direct damage to sweat glands caused by GL-3 deposits and reduced sweat gland innervation (16). The sympathetic skin response may be used to test for sweat gland function but it has a low sensitivity and can appear normal even when sudomotor function is substantially disrupted. This was the case with our patient.

Pain in Fabry disease

In children, pain is often the earliest sign of Fabry disease. The typical manifestation is burning acral pain associated with febrile illnesses. The burning pain in the hands and feet is classically referred to as acroparesthesia although this term is technically incorrect because paresthesia is defined as a non-painful abnormal skin sensation (17). The diagnosis is often missed because the pain is attributed to the infectious illness itself. Later in life, patients may suffer from pain of similar characteristics after physical exertion which can be debilitating. Recurrent, very severe attacks of pain ("pain crises") often begin in the distal extremities and may radiate proximally. They can be so intense that the patient is confined to bed and prescribed opioids. These pain crises may be triggered by a rapidly changing core body temperature, sudden exposure to cold, rapid changes in humidity, and fatigue. As patients age, pain attacks can become less frequent and less intense. Given the lack of clinical trials specifically testing analgesics in Fabry disease, general guidelines for the treatment of neuropathic pain are recommended. Open trials and case histories report successful treatment with phenytoin, carbamazepine, and gabapentin (18–20). The detection of neuropathic pain in Fabry disease is, therefore, important for the following reasons: 1. In children, neuropathic pain may be the first clue to suggest the diagnosis. 2. An early diagnosis can prevent irreversible damage and limit organ involvement (21). 3. The correct diagnosis of neuropathic pain is required to initiate adequate symptomatic therapy and to improve the patient's quality of life.

References

(1) Zarate YA, Hopkin RJ. Fabry's disease. *Lancet* 2008; 372:1427–1435.

(2) Von Korff M, Ormel J, Keefe FJ, Dworkin SF. Grading the severity of chronic pain. *Pain* 1992;40:133–149.

(3) Fellgiebel A. Stroke and brain structural alterations in Fabry disease. *Clin Ther* 2007;29(Suppl A):S9–S10.

(4) Fellgiebel A, Müller MJ, Ginsberg L. CNS manifestations of Fabry's disease. *Lancet Neurol* 2006;5:791–795.

(5) Crutchfield KE, Patronas NJ, Dambrosia JM, et al. Quantitative analysis of cerebral vasculopathy in patients with Fabry disease. *Neurology* 1998;50: 1746–1749.

(6) Lacomis D. Small-fiber neuropathy. *Muscle Nerve* 2002;26:173–188.

(7) Moller AT, Jensen TS. Neurological manifestations in Fabry's disease. *Nat Clin Pract Neurol* 2007;3:95–106.

(8) Torvin Møller A, Winther Bach F, Feldt-Rasmussen U, et al. Functional and structural nerve fiber findings in heterozygote patients with Fabry disease. *Pain* 2009;145:237–245.

(9) Maag R, Binder A, Maier C, et al. Detection of a characteristic painful neuropathy in Fabry disease: a pilot study. *Pain Med* 2008;9:1217–1223.

(10) Rolke R, Baron R, Maier C, et al. Quantitative sensory testing in the German Research Network on Neuropathic Pain (DFNS): standardized protocol and reference values. *Pain* 2006;123:231–243.

(11) Hilz MJ. Evaluation of peripheral and autonomic nerve function in Fabry disease. *Acta Paediatr Suppl* 2002;91:38–42.

(12) Dutsch M, Marthol H, Stemper B, Brys M, Haendl T, Hilz MJ. Small fiber dysfunction predominates in Fabry neuropathy. *J Clin Neurophysiol* 2002;19:575–586.

(13) Luciano CA, Russell JW, Banerjee TK, et al. Physiological characterization of neuropathy in Fabry's disease. *Muscle Nerve* 2002;26:622–629.

(14) Schiffmann R, Floeter MK, Dambrosia JM, et al. Enzyme replacement therapy improves peripheral nerve and sweat function in Fabry disease. *Muscle Nerve* 2003;28:703–710.

(15) Hilz MJ, Brys M, Marthol H, Stemper B, Dutsch M. Enzyme replacement therapy improves function of C-, Adelta-, and Abeta-nerve fibers in Fabry neuropathy. *Neurology* 2004;62:1066–1072.

(16) Yamamoto K, Sobue G, Iwase S, Kumazawa K, Mitsuma T, Mano T. Possible mechanism of anhidrosis in a symptomatic female carrier of Fabry's disease: an assessment by skin sympathetic nerve activity and sympathetic skin response. *Clin Auton Res* 1996;6:107–110.

(17) Weidemann F, Strotmann JM, Breunig F, et al. Misleading terms in Anderson-Fabry disease. *Eur J Clin Invest* 2008;38:191–196.

(18) Duperrat B, Puissant A, Saurat JH, Delanoe MJ, Doyard PA, Grunfeld JP. [Proceedings: Fabry's disease, angiokeratomas present at birth. Effect of diphenylhydantoin on painful attacks]. *Ann Dermatol Syphiligr (Paris)* 1975;102:392–393.

(19) Ries M, Mengel E, Kutschke G, et al. Use of gabapentin to reduce chronic neuropathic pain in Fabry disease. *J Inherit Metab Dis* 2003;26:413–414.

(20) Filling-Katz MR, Merrick HF, Fink JK, Miles RB, Sokol J, Barton NW. Carbamazepine in Fabry's disease: effective analgesia with dose-dependent exacerbation of autonomic dysfunction. *Neurology* 1989;39:598–600.

(21) Desnick RJ, Brady R, Barranger J, et al. Fabry disease, an under-recognized multisystemic disorder: expert recommendations for diagnosis, management, and enzyme replacement therapy. *Ann Intern Med* 2003;138:338–346.

17

Pain and proximal myotonic myopathy (DM2)

Many types of muscle disease can be associated with chronic pain. While these do not classically involve sensory systems, muscles include a large complement of C unmyelinated nociceptive afferents. This vignette describes a patient with myotonic dystrophy Type 2, an autosomal muscular dystrophy with a peculiar predilection for muscle pain.

Clinical case vignette

A 50-year-old man presented with a 24-year history of difficulties with his muscles. Despite a career of professional dancing, he noted difficulty going up stairs and stiffness and slowness of his muscles to "warm up." Five years after the onset of his complaints (19 years earlier, age 31) he could run up a flight of stairs, but at the time of evaluation he was barely able to climb stairs. He had difficulty releasing his grip after holding onto things. He also had prominent pain in the legs, hands, and arms and rated its severity as 6–9/10. The pain was brought on almost immediately after exertion and he could only walk a maximum of two blocks. He also noted some slurring of speech, impaired swallowing of fluids, and difficulty chewing. He had noticed a decline in his balance.

Neurological review was otherwise negative. He had used intravenous street drugs once 30 years earlier and smoked occasional marijuana. He was unable to tolerate mexiletine, phenytoin, or quinine.

He had a family history of neuromuscular disease involving his sister and his son. Other details of the family history were uncertain. His son, aged 28, had a life-long history of "shaky" hands, difficulty releasing things with his hands, and muscle pain on exertion. The son had temporalis and masseter atrophy with atypical clinical percussion myotonia but no muscle weakness. A muscle biopsy in this family member identified only nonspecific changes with rare thin muscle fibers and molecular testing for the DM gene was negative. Medications for his son's pain

included cyclobenzaprine, quinine, amitriptyline, marijuana, baclofen, mexilitene, and gabapentin all with limited benefits or side-effects.

The patient's sister, age 42, had a 20-year history of diffuse limb pain, muscle spasms, and fatigue. She described painful spasms at her hips and knees that would awaken her from sleep. She smoked marijuana and took opioid medications for her pain. She had weakness of proximal muscles without clinical myotonia. Her difficulties progressed over 3 years of follow-up and she developed diffuse wasting, increased proximal limb weakness, neck extensor weakness, and clinical myotonia. She also developed cardiomyopathy and suffered a ventricular thrombus.

On neurological examination of the index patient, he had mild hand incoordination, minimal weakness on arising from a squatting position, and absent ankle reflexes. Muscle strength in both axial and truncal muscles was otherwise intact. He did not exhibit typical percussion myotonia of his thenar muscles.

Electrophysiological studies indicated borderline distal slowing of motor and sensory conduction. Needle electromyography identified myotonic discharges that were recorded in tibialis anterior, vastus medialis, triceps, first dorsal interosseous, biceps, and deltoid muscles. Some of the voluntarily recruited motor unit potentials were decreased in duration and polyphasic, suggestive of a myopathic process. His CK level was mildly elevated at 575 U/L (normal, <195). Hemogram, sedimentation rate, electrolytes (including calcium and magnesium levels), hepatic function, ANA, and TSH level were all normal. A right quadriceps muscle biopsy showed mild nondiagnostic changes: increased central nuclei, excess variation in fiber size with some atrophic muscle fibers, and occasional pyknotic nuclear clumps.

An initial diagnosis of myotonic muscular dystrophy was considered but testing for the DM (DM1) gene variable length polymorphism region was negative. After the family history was established, a clinical diagnosis of autosomal dominant proximal myotonic myopathy, or Myotonic Dystrophy Type 2 (DM2), was made. This was confirmed by identifying a CCTG repeat expansion in the ZNF9 gene. At 7 years following the original evaluation, he had noted a decline in balance and speech and was using a motorized wheelchair outside of the home. He could walk up to 3–4 blocks but usually was exhausted after half a block. He reported continued spasms and pain, rated as 4/10 on average but as severe as 8/10. For his pain, he was using long-acting morphine (130 mg twice daily), extra short-acting morphine for breakthrough pain, and baclofen. On examination he had mild proximal (4+/5 MRC) weakness of deltoids, hip flexors, and quadriceps, intact power otherwise, no myotonia, and mild dysarthria.

Pain description

The pain was described as muscular aching and cramping involving the hands, arms, and legs. The pain was typically worsened from exertion. It was perhaps aggravated by the cold but its onset was unrelated to meals. The intensity of the discomfort could vary. He also experienced chronic neck and lower back discomfort. His son described similar soreness and aching in his legs. His sister also described muscle pains requiring long-term marijuana and opioid use.

Discussion

DM2 is an autosomal dominant disorder of muscles caused by an unstable expansion of a CCTG tetraplet repeat in intron 1 of the zinc finger 9 (ZFN9) gene on chromosome 3q21.3 (1). It is uncertain how the genetic abnormality accounts for the clinical phenotype of the disorder. This patient, his son, and sister (and possibly his father) were similarly involved. Like the better known disorder myotonic dystrophy Type 1 (DM1 or DM), patients with DM2 may develop muscle weakness, stiffness from abnormal excitability of muscles (myotonia), and have abnormalities of other organs such as the brain (e.g., cognitive dysfunction), eyes (cataracts), and the endocrine system (insulin resistance). DM2 is associated with less weakness than DM1, and it predominantly involves proximal muscles (it has also been called PROMM-proximal myotonic myopathy). As in our patient, clinical myotonia is less readily demonstrated but electrical myotonia on needle electromyography may be prominent. CK levels can be mildly elevated and muscle biopsy shows non-

Table 17.1 Pain localization in type 2 diabetes mellitus (DM2)*

Pain variable[†]	Patients with DM2/PROMM	Patients with OMD
Limb muscles: Proximal	22/24	13/24
Distal	20/24	13/24
Arms	17/24[‡]	7/24
Forearms	12/24	6/24
Hands/fingers	4/24	6/24
Thighs	19/24[‡]	9/24
Lower legs	17/24	12/24
Calf	13/24	11/24
Anterior tibial muscle	11/24[§]	0/24
Peroneal	3/24	1/24
Feet	5/24	6/24
Limb girdles:	15/24	8/24
Low back:	17/24	10/24
Others: Knee	8/24	2/24
Jaw	3/24	2/24
Unilateral:	4/24	3/24
Bilateral: Asymmetrical	1/24	5/24
Symmetrical	20/24	16/24
Radiating pain	14/24[§]	0/24

*Radiating, pain radiating from the pelvic limb girdle to the thighs or lower legs. Details of pain description from George et al. (2) in DM2, including its localization, site, and radiation (a) and its descriptors (b) using the McGill pain questionnaire.
[†]Data were obtained with MPQ. Data indicate the number of patients with this variable out of the total number of patients examined.
[‡]Significantly different from OMD ($P < 0.05$; Fisher's exact test).
[§]Significantly different from OMD ($P < 0.001$; Fisher's exact test).

specific alterations. Unlike DM1, pain is a prominent feature of DM2.

Pain in DM2

Pain is a common feature of DM2, reported to occur in 46% of patients (1, 2). Its presence is unrelated to the presence or severity of myotonia and it may render discomfort to touch or muscle palpation. Some patients may have chest pain that is mistaken for cardiac disease. Nonetheless, DM2 is also associated with cardiac conduction abnormalities, but less frequently than in DM1. While our patient had pain brought on by exercise, the pain in DM2 may not necessarily be exercise related.

George et al. (2) identified musculoskeletal pain in 23 of 24 patients with DM2 in their clinic. Their mean age was 57 and symptoms of muscle disease had been present for a mean of 15 years. The pain was localized to muscles and several types of pain were described (mean of 5 and a maximum of 12 pain types/patient). The pain rating index using the McGill pain questionnaire and the numbers of pain types were greater in DM2 patients than those with other muscular disorders. Descriptors included "tugging," "dull," "stabbing," "sore," "tender," and "exhausting." Pain was proximal and distal involving arms, forearms, thighs, and lower legs most often. Feet and hands were less involved and the pain was often described as asymmetrical. In 8 patients, musculoskeletal pain was the most disabling feature of their condition compared with 3 of 24 patients with other muscular disorders. Pain was frequently exacerbated by exercise (17/24 patients), by cold (10/24), or by palpation (11/24). Pain also usually persisted for 6 months or more. The findings did not support the use of massage for treatment, an approach that worsened symptoms. Overall the findings identified a unique pain phenotype differing from that of patients with other muscle disorders. Summary information from this source is illustrated in Table 17.1.

The mechanism of pain in DM2 is unknown. It is described as deep and cramping despite the finding that myotonia and cramps in DM2 are much less common than in DM1 where pain is infrequent. It is interesting that both in our patient and his sister, several analgesics were tried with mixed results. Our patient found some mild benefit from mexilitene. Both brother and sister found smoking marijuana helped their symptoms. Ischemic and overcontracted muscles can generate intense pain in patients likely through the participation of a rich unmyelinated nociceptor population that innervates muscles. A separate genetic alteration of sensory axon function in DM2 cannot be excluded. DM2 pain is chronic and not associated with muscle fiber necrosis, yet it localizes to both limb and truncal muscles suggesting an interaction between deep afferents and abnormal muscle molecular architecture. No specific forms of treatment have been identified for DM2.

References

(1) Meola G, Moxley RT, III. Myotonic dystrophy type 2 and related myotonic disorders. *J Neurol* 2004;251: 1173–1182.

(2) George A, Schneider-Gold C, Zier S, Reiners K, Sommer C. Musculoskeletal pain in patients with myotonic dystrophy type 2. *Arch Neurol* 2004;61: 1938–1942.

Chapter

18

Complex regional pain syndrome

Complex regional pain syndromes (CRPS), encompassing previous terms such as causalgia, reflex sympathetic dystrophy, Sudeck's atrophy, and others, complicate soft tissue or peripheral nerve damage to an extremity. It is a challenging pain syndrome both for the patient and the clinician.

Clinical case vignette

A 52-year-old, right-handed truck driver fell from his truck while unloading some goods. He noticed pain and swelling of his left hand and pain at his left hip and left ankle. Despite his injuries, he drove approximately 500 km to his home. He visited the local hospital 2 days after the accident. The examining physician found a grossly swollen left hand but an x-ray revealed no fracture. Two days later, the pain and swelling had not subsided and the patient visited a second physician. A distal radius fracture was diagnosed. An open cast was applied to the left lower arm. The patient was re-examined 5 days later. Blood supply and sensory and motor function in the arm were found to be normal and a circular cast was applied. The patient rated his pain as 2 on a scale of 0–10.

The cast was removed 6 weeks later. Shortly thereafter, the patient reported a massive increase in pain, up to 8/10. He felt mild pain at rest (3/10) but the slightest hand movement, such as during physiotherapy, exacerbated the pain. His physician noted swelling and a slight bluish discoloration of the left hand. There was a decreased range of motion of the fingers and wrist. Range of motion at the wrist was reduced to extension of 40° and flexion of 70°. The patient reported that the swelling was variable, and that the color of the hand could change from bluish to deep red. He was treated with acupuncture and transcutaneous electrotherapy for 3 months by his orthopedic surgeon, but his condition did not improve. When the patient tried to move his hand, his pain ratings increased to 8/10. Because movement was still

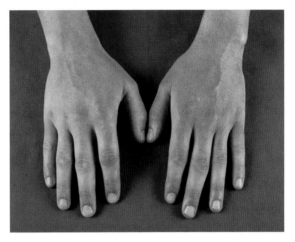

Figure 18.1. Mild CRPS of the left hand with discoloration (red), edema, and prominent veins.

restricted, a repeat radiograph was performed which showed spotty osteoporotic changes at the trapezius and the base of the first metacarpal bone. The patient was referred to a specialist for hand surgery at which point a diagnosis of CRPS I was established.

Approximately 6 months following the initial injury, the patient obtained appointments at a pain clinic. Swelling of the left hand with disturbed vaso- and sudomotor function were noted. The left hand felt warmer to touch, and sweating was increased [Figure 18.1]. Motor strength was reduced due to pain. Repeated sympathetic blocks of the stellate ganglion were performed twice weekly for 5 weeks. Under this treatment, pain at rest resolved and pain with movements was reduced to 4–5/10. The range of motion increased. An attempt to further improve the situation by combining the treatment with 25 mg of amitriptyline at bedtime was unsuccessful because of anticholinergic side-effects. A selective serotonin reuptake inhibitor, citalopram, was then prescribed but discontinued because of nervous agitation.

During the following months, the patient received regular physiotherapy. His condition was stable but he was not pain free, particularly when moving the left hand. Approximately 1 year after the initial injury, the patient underwent hip replacement surgery on the right. In this context, he received a course of bisphosphonates after which he reported his left hand to be pain free. Notably, within 1 month of using crutches for mobility, pain in the left hand recurred with strength of 6/10. Sympathetic blocks and intravenous application of bisphosphonates were repeated. Follow-up examinations revealed that the patient was pain-free most of the time. He felt intermittent exacerbations of pain after exertion or sometimes spontaneously that usually resolved within several days. Except for evidence of a reduced callus on the left, no difference between the hands were noted on inspection, and skin temperature was equal on both sides. The range of movement was normal. Left grip strength was still reduced compared with the right. Nerve conduction studies of the ulnar, median, and radial nerve were normal.

Pain description

During the acute phase of his CRPS, the patient described pain at rest and upon moving the hand. His pain at rest had a severity of 3–4/10 and upon movement its severity could increase to 8/10. After using the left hand, pain at rest worsened for periods of several hours to days. Also, swelling and discoloration of the hand also increased following exertion. As a result, the patient tended to restrict use of his left hand. When describing the pain, the patient used descriptors like aching, stabbing, sharp, and sometimes burning.

Discussion

This patient had a typical, moderately severe course of CRPS I. His pain increased when it should have abated. Swelling, discoloration, temperature changes, sweating disturbances, and motor dysfunction were present (see Figure 18.1 for an example from a different patient). The course was protracted, symptoms improved with treatment and with time, and exacerbations occurred upon increased use of the hand. Finally, the patient reached a stable, almost pain-free state. Treatment in this patient was challenging and alternative approaches may have been more effective.

Most physicians cite the publication, "Gunshot wounds and other injuries of nerves" by Mitchell (1)

in the middle of the 19th century as the first description of CRPS. It was then termed causalgia due to the burning character of the pain. At the beginning of the 20th century, Paul Sudeck, a surgeon from Hamburg, Germany, published a study about posttraumatic bone atrophy (2) describing a pain syndrome associated with edema and trophic changes of the skin. Later, the term sympathetic reflex dystrophy was coined because clinical investigations revealed that the disorder appeared to be caused by overactivity of the sympathetic nervous system; sympathetic blocks were believed effective analgesic agents (3). When later studies raised doubts about the reflexive activation of the sympathetic nervous system, the International Association for the Study of Pain (IASP) introduced a purely descriptive term, complex regional pain syndrome (CRPS). This remains the official term for this syndrome (4).

Traditionally, CRPS is classified as CRPS I and CRPS II. In CRPS I, there is no overt nerve injury, in CRPS II, there is injury of a major nerve trunk. Because injury of small nerves and nerve endings occurs in all trauma, the distinction has recently been debated (5), in particular because reduced skin innervation has also been shown in CRPS I (6, 7).

As with many disorders involving pain, CRPS is confirmed by specific diagnostic criteria (8). These "Budapest criteria" are reproduced in Table 18.1. Pain, disproportionate to the inciting event, is obligatory. Edema, discoloration, and other vasomotor abnormalities may vary in intensity as described in Figure 18.1. Trophic changes may occur in approximately 50% of patients. These include increased hair- and nail growth in the acute stage, but reduced hair- and nail growth and skin atrophy in chronic stages. Severely affected patients may also develop muscle atrophy and contractures.

Approximately 75% of patients have weakness of the involved site (9). In acute stages, this may be pain-dependent and guarding may result. Range of motion may be reduced due to edema. In chronic stages, contractions and fibrosis on palmar and plantar sides of hands or feet may impede movement. Tremor, myoclonus, and dystonia may occur, increasing in frequency in chronic cases (9, 10).

Pain in CRPS

Apart from the clinical distinction between CRPS I (without major nerve trunk injury) and CRPS II (with

Table 18.1 Clinical diagnostic criteria for CRPS according to Harden et al. (27)

1. Persisting pain, which is disproportionate to any inciting event

2. At least one symptom in three of the four following categories:
   Sensory symptoms: reports of hyperesthesia and/or allodynia
   Vasomotor symptoms: reports of temperature asymmetry and/or skin color changes and/or skin color asymmetry
   Sudomotor/edema symptoms: reports of edema and/or sweating changes and/or sweating asymmetry
   Motor/trophic symptoms: reports of decreased range of motion and/or motor dysfunction (weakness, tremor, dystonia) and/or trophic changes (hair, nail, skin)

3. At least one sign demonstrated in two or more of the following categories at time of evaluation:
   Sensory signs: evidence of hyperalgesia (to pinprick) and/or allodynia (to light touch and/or deep somatic pressure and/or joint movement)
   Vasomotor signs: evidence of temperature asymmetry and/or skin color changes and/or asymmetry
   Sudomotor/edema signs: evidence of edema and/or sweating changes and/or sweating asymmetry
   Motor/trophic signs: evidence of decreased range of motion and/or motor dysfunction (weakness, tremor, dystonia) and/or trophic changes (hair, nail, skin)

4. There is no other diagnosis that better explains the signs and symptoms

nerve injury), patients may also be described as having "warm" or "cold" CRPS. The warm type usually develops post-traumatically, the skin is red and skin temperature is increased on the affected side. If the disorder becomes chronic, the skin may acquire bluish overtones and become cold. The cold phenotype is rare (20%) and often develops following minor trauma or even spontaneously (5).

Most patients with CRPS have pain at rest (11). It is often perceived as deep pain although it may also consist of a superficial sensation on the skin. It is described as tearing, burning, or stinging. Numbness, paresthesias, or a feeling of foreignness of the affected limb occurs in up to 30% of patients. Nearly all patients report increased pain under certain circumstances, for example when lowering the limb, upon joint movement, or upon light touch. Brush-evoked pain (cutaneous dynamic mechanical allodynia) is present in approximately 30% of CRPS patients and is more common in the chronic phase.

Quantitative sensory testing reveals hyperalgesia to pressure, but somewhat paradoxically, deficits in the perception of cold and warm as well as vibratory stimuli (12) [Figure 18.2].

The pathophysiology of CRPS is incompletely understood (13). Several contributing factors however, have been identified. Following injury, peripheral neurogenic inflammation occurs with release of inflammatory mediators like neuropeptides-cytokines, and growth factors (5, 12, 14). This process is reversed during normal healing, but persists in CRPS. Consequently, some researchers regard CRPS as a deficiency in resolution of inflammation. A genetic component may also be involved, although only a few gene polymorphisms related to CRPS have been identified, i.e., the HLA system in patients with CRPS and dystonia (15). Associations with other candidate genes are inconclusive. During the process of injury and inflammation, cutaneous innervation is damaged (6) with deficits in cutaneous sensitivity (12). This may contribute to trophic skin changes. The sympathetic innervation can be equally involved. Similar processes likely occur in the deep tissues but this has not been confirmed. Continuous afferent input from damaged and sensitized nociceptors may then lead to plasticity in the central pain pathways as confirmed by functional imaging studies of the brain, electrophysiological brain mapping, and receptor-ligand studies (13, 16). All changes appear reversible whether due to natural healing processes or following treatment of the condition (17).

Systemic corticosteroids can be effective if prescribed early in the disease process (18, 19). The usual dose is 30–40 mg/day of prednisolone-equivalent for 4 weeks, or 1 mg/kg for 1 week with tapering over 3 weeks. Bisphosphonates have been successful as demonstrated in four controlled trials (alendronate (20, 21), clodronate (22), pamidronate (23)). They reduce pain, improve function, and block osteoclast activity. Data on calcitonin are discrepant. Case reports confirm some success with intravenous immunoglobulin and TNF blockers. Topical dimethylsulfoxide (DMSO 50%), a free-radical scavenger, may also have benefit (24). Physiotherapy and ergotherapy are recommended, but should be performed by a therapist with special knowledge of CRPS to prevent complications. Motor imagery (mirror therapy) may be efficient (25). It is important that the patients

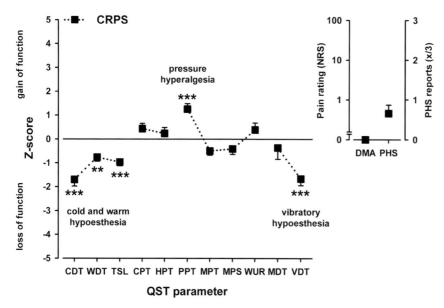

Figure 18.2. Example of results of quantitative sensory testing in a cohort of CRPS patients. Reproduced with permission from Üçeyler et al. (12). Z-score sensory profile of 31 CRPS patients on the affected limb. The Z-score profile of CRPS patients was compared with healthy control subjects as represented by a Z-score "zero." The sensory profile of the affected limbs shows a predominant loss of sensory function in terms of cold hypoesthesia (CDT), warm hypoesthesia (WDT), an increased threshold for the detection of temperature differences (thermal sensory limen, TSL), an increased number of paradoxical heat sensations (PHS), and vibratory hypoesthesia (VDT). In contrast to a decreased cutaneous sensitivity across C-fiber, A-delta- and A-beta-fiber mediated stimuli, deep pain sensitivity to blunt pressure (PPT) was increased. This sensory profile is consistent with deafferentation in combination with peripheral sensitization of the nociceptive system in this subgroup of CRPS patients. Z-score: Numbers of standard deviations between patient data and group-specific mean values of healthy control subjects. MPT: mechanical pain threshold; MPS: mechanical pain sensitivity; WUR: wind-up ratio; MDT: mechanical detection threshold; VDT: vibration detection threshold; DMA: dynamic mechanical allodynia. Shown data represent mean Z-scores ± SEM. For DMA and PHS raw data are shown (mean ± SEM). $*P < 0.05$; $**P < 0.01$; $***P < 0.001$ (one-way analysis of variance).

practice these therapies independently between regular guided sessions. Sympathetic blocks can be used when less invasive measures prove insufficient. Spinal cord stimulation or intrathecal baclofen may be an option for patients with otherwise refractory pain (26). Psychotherapy is indicated if there are psychological comorbidities such as depression and anxiety.

References

(1) Mitchell SW, Morehouse GR, Keen WW. *Gunshot Wounds and Other Injuries of Nerves.* Philadelphia: JB Lippincott & Co., 1864.

(2) Sudeck P. Über die akute (reflektorische) Knochenatrophie nach Entzündungen und Verletzungen in den Extremitäten und ihre klinischen Erscheinungen. *Fortschr Röntgenstr* 1901;5:227–293.

(3) Bonica JJ. Causalgia and other reflex sympathetic dystrophies. In: Bonica JJ, ed. *Advances in Pain Research and Therapy.* New York: Raven Press, 1979:141–166.

(4) Merskey H, Bogduk N. *Classification of Chronic Pain. Descriptions of Chronic Pain Syndromes and Definition of Pain Terms.* Seattle: IASP Press, 1994.

(5) Birklein F. Complex regional pain syndrome. In: Aminoff MJ, Boller F, Swaab DF, eds. *Handbook of Clinical Neurology.* Edinburgh: Elsevier, 2006:529–546.

(6) Albrecht PJ, Hines S, Eisenberg E, et al. Pathologic alterations of cutaneous innervation and vasculature in affected limbs from patients with complex regional pain syndrome. *Pain* 2006;120:244–266.

(7) Oaklander AL, Fields HL. Is reflex sympathetic dystrophy/complex regional pain syndrome type I a small-fiber neuropathy? *Ann Neurol* 2009;65:629–638.

(8) Harden RN, Bruehl S, Perez RS, et al. Validation of proposed diagnostic criteria (the "Budapest Criteria") for Complex Regional Pain Syndrome. *Pain* 2010; 150:268–274.

(9) de Boer RD, Marinus J, van Hilten JJ, et al. Distribution of signs and symptoms of complex regional pain syndrome type I in patients meeting the

diagnostic criteria of the International Association for the Study of Pain. *Eur J Pain* 2011;15:830.e1-8.

(10) van Hilten JJ. Movement disorders in complex regional pain syndrome. *Pain Med* 2010;11: 1274–1277.

(11) Birklein F, Riedl B, Sieweke N, Weber M, Neundorfer B. Neurological findings in complex regional pain syndromes–analysis of 145 cases. *Acta Neurol Scand* 2000;101:262–269.

(12) Üçeyler N, Eberle T, Rolke R, Birklein F, Sommer C. Differential expression patterns of cytokines in complex regional pain syndrome. *Pain* 2007;132: 195–205.

(13) Bruehl S. An update on the pathophysiology of complex regional pain syndrome. *Anesthesiology* 2010;113:713–725.

(14) Krämer HH, Eberle T, Üçeyler N, et al. TNF-alpha in CRPS and "normal" trauma – significant differences between tissue and serum. *Pain* 2011;152:285–290.

(15) de Rooij AM, Florencia Gosso M, Haasnoot GW, et al. HLA-B62 and HLA-DQ8 are associated with Complex Regional Pain Syndrome with fixed dystonia. *Pain* 2009;145:82–85.

(16) Klega A, Eberle T, Buchholz HG, et al. Central opioidergic neurotransmission in complex regional pain syndrome. *Neurology* 2010;75:129–136.

(17) Maihofner C, Handwerker HO, Neundorfer B, Birklein F. Cortical reorganization during recovery from complex regional pain syndrome. *Neurology* 2004;63:693–701.

(18) Christensen K, Jensen EM, Noer I. The reflex dystrophy syndrome response to treatment with systemic corticosteroids. *Acta Chir Scand* 1982; 148:653–655.

(19) Kalita J, Vajpayee A, Misra UK. Comparison of prednisolone with piroxicam in complex regional

pain syndrome following stroke: a randomized controlled trial. *QJM* 2006;99:89–95.

(20) Adami S, Fossaluzza V, Gatti D, Fracassi E, Braga V. Bisphosphonate therapy of reflex sympathetic dystrophy syndrome. *Ann Rheum Dis* 1997;56: 201–204.

(21) Manicourt DH, Brasseur JP, Boutsen Y, Depreseux G, Devogelaer JP. Role of alendronate in therapy for posttraumatic complex regional pain syndrome type I of the lower extremity. *Arthritis Rheum* 2004;50: 3690–3697.

(22) Varenna M, Zucchi F, Ghiringhelli D, et al. Intravenous clodronate in the treatment of reflex sympathetic dystrophy syndrome. A randomized, double blind, placebo controlled study. *J Rheumatol* 2000;27:1477–1483.

(23) Robinson JN, Sandom J, Chapman PT. Efficacy of pamidronate in complex regional pain syndrome type I. *Pain Med* 2004;5:276–280.

(24) Zuurmond WW, Langendijk PN, Bezemer PD, Brink HE, de Lange JJ, van Loenen AC. Treatment of acute reflex sympathetic dystrophy with DMSO 50% in a fatty cream. *Acta Anaesthesiol Scand* 1996;40:364–367.

(25) Moseley GL, Zalucki N, Birklein F, Marinus J, van Hilten JJ, Luomajoki H. Thinking about movement hurts: the effect of motor imagery on pain and swelling in people with chronic arm pain. *Arthritis Rheum* 2008;59:623–631.

(26) Tran de QH, Duong S, Bertini P, Finlayson RJ. Treatment of complex regional pain syndrome: a review of the evidence. *Can J Anaesth* 2010;57: 149–166.

(27) Harden RN, Bruehl S, Stanton-Hicks M, Wilson PR. Proposed new diagnostic criteria for complex regional pain syndrome. *Pain Med* 2007;8: 326–331.

Pain and polymyalgia rheumatica

Polymyalgia rheumatica is a subacute disorder that may be associated with deep aching proximal muscle weakness. We describe a patient with this disorder who was initially considered to have an inflammatory myopathy.

Clinical case vignette

A 75-year-old man was evaluated after a 5- to 6-month history of pain and limb weakness. He had difficulty arising from a toilet or low chair and required hand support to ascend stairs. Muscle pain was prominent in his thighs and hips, limiting his ability to use farm machinery. He noticed some improvement when he took doses of his wife's non-steroidal anti-inflammatory medication. He also noticed some mild right temporomandibular joint discomfort with chewing but denied rash, dysphagia, neck weakness, diploplia, or change in speech. There were no headaches or visual changes. He had lost 10 kg in weight and thought there was atrophy of his thighs. In the past, he had suffered knee osteoarthritis, coronary artery disease, and hyperlipidemia. He had a brother with polymyalgia rheumatica and a nephew with amyotrophic lateral sclerosis (ALS).

On neurological examination, he had normal extraocular movements and neck muscle power. There was mild and questionable proximal upper limb weakness, and mild deltoid and quadriceps loss of bulk. He could not arise from a squat or chair without using his arms. Deep tendon reflexes and sensation were intact.

He had been started on two doses of prednisone 50 mg 6 days before evaluation which was then discontinued until the time of neurological evaluation. His ESR was borderline elevated at 14 (normal, <10 mm/h), C-reactive protein elevated at 20.8 (normal, < 8.0 mg/L), and CK normal. Other blood work was normal, including electrolytes, quantitative RF, ANA screen, SSA/Ro, and TSH. Electrophysiological studies were largely normal, including repetitive

conduction studies. Needle electromyography identified minor changes in motor unit configuration (small amplitude and duration MUPs) in right deltoid and triceps, but there was no abnormal spontaneous activity. Iliopsoas was normal. A left deltoid muscle biopsy was normal and a diagnosis of polymyalgia rheumatica (PMR) was made. He resumed prednisone after the muscle biopsy with a gradual tapering course from 50 mg daily over the next 3 months. At that time, he reported dramatic improvement in his pain and muscle function. Neurological examination indicated that he had normal muscle power throughout and no difficulty arising from a chair without use of his arms. He had regained weight.

Pain description

The patient described deep aching proximal muscle pain largely centered around his "hips" and thighs. The pain interfered with his ability to work and climb stairs, and it responded dramatically to the use of glucocorticoid therapy.

Discussion

PMR is an auto-immune inflammatory disorder that presents in older patients with proximal muscle pain and weakness. Although patients describe weakness, formal neurological examination is either normal or, as in the patient described here, demonstrates equivocal weakness. Apparent weakness may be secondary to pain and limited voluntary effort. Morning "stiffness" is frequently described. Important negatives are the absence of ophthalmoparesis, neck flexor weakness, or extensor weakness. The patients have intact reflexes and sensation. PMR is associated with temporal arteritis, not diagnosed in the patient described here despite some very mild temporomandibular joint discomfort. A high index of suspicion however, is required in patients with PMR to identify temporal arteritis given the serious risks of visual loss. Rarely patients may suffer cerebral infarction from giant cell arterial damage. Additional clinical features accompanying PMR include weight loss, occasional fever, and anemia. Our patient had weight loss but did not develop anemia. Key laboratory diagnostic features are elevation of the ESR (>40 mm/h) and CRP. Whereas only the CRP was significantly elevated in our patient, he had received two doses of oral prednisone before his evaluation that may have partly treated his PMR. Electrophysiological studies are characteristically normal or may show borderline changes in motor unit configuration. Muscle biopsy may be normal or occasionally shows nonspecific changes such as "moth-eaten" fibers. The biopsy in PMR does not identify inflammation. Finally, the clinical response to steroid is a key feature; dramatic improvement, as in the patient described here, is expected. Most instances of PMR are sporadic, and the description of PMR in his brother is unusual.

While our patient initially received high doses of prednisone, recent evidence-based reviews suggest that a dose of 15 mg is appropriate and reduces the risks of long-term prednisone-related side-effects (1). Methotrexate (e.g., 10 mg/wk) can be offered as a steroid sparing agent. Because relapses can occur, therapy for up to 2 years may be required.

Pain in polymyalgia rheumatica

The mechanisms of proximal muscle pain that develop in PMR patients are uncertain, given the nonspecific muscle biopsy findings. Activation of deep muscle or connective tissue unmyelinated C-fibers by inflammatory cytokines or limited ischemic damage from arteritis are possibilities. Kreiner and Galbo described elevated cytokines in PMR that included interleukin-1β (IL-1β), IL-1 receptor antagonist, IL-6, IL-8, and monocyte chemoattractant protein 1. In a separate report, these authors also noted elevated glutamate and PGE (2) within muscle in PMR patients compared with control or patient plasma levels (2, 3). Shintani et al. (4) observed elevated IgG, IgA, and fibrinogen deposits in the perifascicular area of the perimysium in patients with PMR. How these rises in cytokines and other molecules are generated and their impact on local pain afferents is uncertain.

References

(1)   Hernandez-Rodriguez J, Cid MC, Lopez-Soto A, Espigol-Frigole G, Bosch X. Treatment of polymyalgia rheumatica: a systematic review. *Arch Intern Med* 2009;169:1839–1850.

(2)   Kreiner F, Galbo H. Elevated muscle interstitial levels of pain-inducing substances in symptomatic muscles in patients with polymyalgia rheumatica. *Pain* 2011;152:1127–1132.

(3)   Kreiner F, Langberg H, Galbo H. Increased muscle interstitial levels of inflammatory cytokines in polymyalgia rheumatica. *Arthritis Rheum* 2010;62: 3768–3775.

(4)   Shintani S, Shiigai T, Matsui Y. Polymyalgia rheumatica (PMR): clinical, laboratory, and immunofluorescence studies in 13 patients. *Clin Neurol Neurosurg* 2002;104:20–29.

Chapter

20

Phantom pain

The enigmatic phenomenon of phantom pain, i.e., pain perceived in a body part that is no longer present, has intrigued physicians and scientists for centuries. This is reflected in the descriptions of numerous case reports in the older literature and more recently, by a series of studies using sophisticated functional brain imaging. The following case report illustrates the challenge but also the possibilities for success when phantom pain is treated in the acute stage.

Clinical case vignette

A 31-year-old engineer presented 4 weeks after amputation of the right leg at the thigh and asked for an invasive procedure to alleviate pain. He described the pain as intermittent, sharp, shooting, and cramp-like. He had developed severe electrifying pain perceived to be in the amputated right foot within days of his surgery. A stump revision 2 weeks later yielded an improvement that lasted for 3 days. Carbamazepine and tilidine/naloxone had been given without success. Infiltration of the stump with the local anesthetic mepivacaine provided pain relief for approximately an hour. Current therapy consisted of diclofenac 50 mg tid, amitriptyline 50 mg tid, and tramadol 75 mg tid. On examination, the stump was bland but painful to touch.

Further history-taking revealed that the patient's right leg had been deformed from birth with a fixed flexion in the knee. The atrophic lower leg extended laterally at an angle of approximately 90° [Figure 20.1]. Despite this malformation, the patient had led a normal life. He was fully integrated in society having completed an engineering degree and he had recently embarked on his career. He had married and had become the father of a healthy daughter. He was active in sports. His motivation for the amputation was twofold; he wanted to wear a prosthesis in his professional environment to avoid attention and on a per-

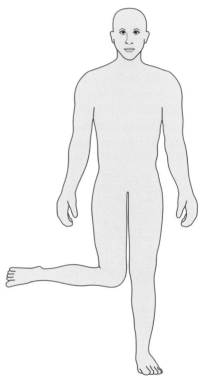

Figure 20.1. A drawing of the patient's deformed lower limb before amputation, based on his description.

sonal note, he wanted to hold his daughter in his arms while standing upright.

The patient was advised about the use of a transcutaneous electrical nerve stimulator (TENS). He was prescribed sustained-release morphine (20 mg bid) under comedication with sodium picosulfate as a laxative, and fast-acting morphine for breakthrough pain (morphine hydrochloride oral solution 2%, up to 20 mg every 6 h). Amitriptyline was increased to 125 mg/day. One week later, the patient reported that TENS had no effect. He had good pain relief for 2–3 h after taking the opiate medication. However, he complained about side-effects, including fatigue, sweating,

Table 20.1. Reported incidence of phantom limb pain in the literature*

Reference	N	% Phantom pain
Ewalt et al., 1947 (22)	2284	2
Henderson and Smyth, 1948 (23)	~300	~1.5
Abramson and Feibel, 1981 (24)	2000	~2
Sherman and Sherman, 1983 (25)	764	85
Sherman et al., 1984 (26)	2750	78
Pohjolainen, 1991 (27)	124	59
Houghton et al., 1994 (2)	176	78
Wartan et al., 1997 (28)	526	55
Kooijman et al., 2000 (29)	124	51
Ephraim et al., 2005 (30)	914	80
Taghipour et al., 2009 (31)	141	89
Kern et al., 2009 (32)	537	75

* Only large case series with >100 patients were considered.

constipation, and hypotension. He was given dihydroergotamine as prolonged-release tablets bid, and a more potent laxative. The patient returned 3 months later and reported of his ability to return to work shortly after the previous visit. He had experienced good pain relief with tolerable side-effects. He had managed to taper his medication to the point of being pain-free without analgesia for 4 weeks. He reported a phantom sensation but it was benign or painless and did not impact his activities.

Pain description

The onset of pain began within days following the amputation. The pain was not constant but intermittent. The sensation was most intense in the missing foot, the patient describing it as electric-shock–like, stabbing, shooting, and sometimes throbbing and boring. Pain attacks could be provoked by pressure to the stump, but also occurred spontaneously. In the acute phase, the patient rated the pain intensity as 10/10. When he was first treated with opioids, the intensity decreased to 5/10 when the drugs achieved their maximum effect.

Discussion

Phantom pain may occur in almost any body part but is most frequently reported after limb amputation. The reported incidence varies considerably

[Table 20.1] due to several factors. It may be difficult to distinguish phantom pain from residual limb pain or from phantom sensation, which is benign in nature. In earlier studies, frequencies were calculated from medical records of patients seeking pain treatment and perhaps underestimated when compared with more recent and objective studies (1). Time after amputation is an important factor determining the prevalence of phantom pain. Most studies show a decrease of phantom pain prevalence over a longer time-frame (2, 3). A study involving 42 patients with amputations for cancer confirmed that 60% had phantom pain at 1 month and 32% at 2 years (4). The severity of phantom pain also appears to decline over time (5, 6).

Seventy-five percent of patients complain of pain onset within the first week after surgery (7). Additionally, there are individual case reports of onset years after amputation. Constant daily pain appears rare in the chronic phase; occurrences between several times per day and less than once a month have been reported (8). The pain often occurs intermittently, and the duration of each attack varies between seconds and hours, rarely days. The pain is mostly localized distally, regardless of the level of amputation. Patients use a wide range of pain descriptors. The pain is variously described as shooting, burning, stabbing, or cramping. Patients may experience electrical shocks, itching, throbbing, and tingling. Phantom pain is occasionally similar to preamputation pain (1).

Many predisposing factors toward the development of phantom pain have been studied. Possible predictors include preamputation pain and acute postoperative pain (9). In a group of patients with lower limb amputation due to peripheral vascular disease, the use of passive coping strategies, especially catastrophizing before amputation, was associated with phantom pain (10).

Phantom pain

Understanding of the pathophysiology of phantom pain is still incomplete. Several studies demonstrate neuroplastic changes in somatosensory and motor cortices following limb amputation (11, 12) [Figure 20.2]. A relationship between the reorganization in the sensory cortex and the intensity of phantom pain has been observed (11). Peripheral causes likely also contribute. Because amputees with chronic residual limb pain have phantom pain more frequently, it has been suggested that neuromas in the stump exhibit abnormal

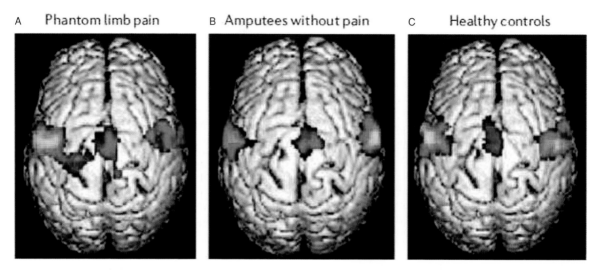

Figure 20.2. Reorganization of the cortex related to phantom pain. (A) Functional MRI data during a lip pursing task. Activation in primary somatosensory and motor cortices in amputees without pain (B) is similar to that of healthy controls (C). In patients with phantom limb pain (A), the cortical representation of the mouth extends into the region of the hand and arm. Reproduced with permission from Oxford University Press (33).

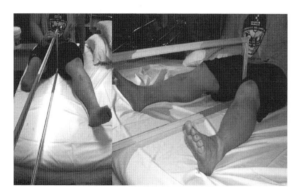

Figure 20.3. Setup for mirror therapy used for a lower limb amputee. Reproduced with permission from Neurologist [1].

activity, triggering the pain. Ramachandran and Hirstein propose at least five different sources of phantom pain: residual limb neuromas, cortical remapping, corollary discharge, body image, and somatic memories, thus linking phantom pain to both cortical and peripheral mechanisms (1).

It has long been debated whether any preventive treatment might be efficacious in phantom pain. A systematic review published in 2010 could not find robust evidence that pre-emptive analgesia minimized the risk of chronic pain after amputation for critical ischemia of peripheral vascular disease (13). Recently, optimized epidural analgesia or intravenous patient-controlled analgesia, initiated 48 h pre-operatively and continuing for 48 h postoperatively, was shown to decrease phantom pain at 6 months in a study with 65 patients (14). Use of a prolonged postoperative perineural infusion of ropivacaine 0.5% yielded a similar effect at 1 year (15). Intense pre-emptive analgesia is consequently recommended before amputation (16).

Once phantom pain occurs, pharmacological and non-pharmacological treatment should be initiated. Many case reports show some improvement with TENS, but a recent meta-analysis could not identify high quality evidence of its efficacy (17). Currently, mirror therapy is regarded as the most promising non-pharmacological therapy for phantom pain (1). Patients see their intact limb reflected in a mirror placed parasagittally between the arms or legs. They are instructed to move the intact limb and the phantom limb simultaneously (18)[Figure 20.1]. Patients have reported a relief of spasm-like phantom pain following a single session (18). A small randomized, sham-controlled, cross-over study conducted in lower limb amputees confirmed a significant impact of mirror therapy (19).

Several drugs have been tested for their efficacy in relieving phantom limb pain. Positive results from randomized controlled trials are available for morphine, amitriptyline and other tricyclic antidepressants (1). Deep brain stimulation (20) and spinal cord stimulation have been used with success in case series of otherwise refractory patients (21).

References

(1) Weeks SR, Anderson-Barnes VC, Tsao JW. Phantom limb pain: theories and therapies. *Neurologist* 2010;16:277–286.

(2) Houghton AD, Nicholls G, Houghton AL, Saadah E, McColl L. Phantom pain: natural history and association with rehabilitation. *Ann R Coll Surg Engl* 1994;76:22–25.

(3) Jensen TS, Krebs B, Nielsen J, Rasmussen P. Immediate and long-term phantom limb pain in amputees: incidence, clinical characteristics and relationship to pre-amputation limb pain. *Pain* 1985;21:267–278.

(4) Mishra S, Bhatnagar S, Gupta D, Diwedi A. Incidence and management of phantom limb pain according to World Health Organization analgesic ladder in amputees of malignant origin. *Am J Hosp Palliat Care* 2007;24:455–462.

(5) Hunter JP, Katz J, Davis KD. Stability of phantom limb phenomena after upper limb amputation: a longitudinal study. *Neuroscience* 2008;156:939–949.

(6) Bosmans JC, Geertzen JH, Post WJ, van der Schans CP, Dijkstra PU. Factors associated with phantom limb pain: a 31/2-year prospective study. *Clin Rehabil* 2010;24:444–453.

(7) Nikolajsen L, Jensen TS. Phantom limb pain. *Br J Anaesth* 2001;87:107–116.

(8) Schley MT, Wilms P, Toepfner S, et al. Painful and nonpainful phantom and stump sensations in acute traumatic amputees. *J Trauma* 2008;65:858–864.

(9) Hanley MA, Jensen MP, Smith DG, Ehde DM, Edwards WT, Robinson LR. Preamputation pain and acute pain predict chronic pain after lower extremity amputation. *J Pain* 2007;8:102–109.

(10) Richardson C, Glenn S, Horgan M, Nurmikko T. A prospective study of factors associated with the presence of phantom limb pain six months after major lower limb amputation in patients with peripheral vascular disease. *J Pain* 2007;8:793–801.

(11) Flor H, Nikolajsen L, Staehelin Jensen T. Phantom limb pain: a case of maladaptive CNS plasticity? *Nat Rev Neurosci* 2006;7:873–881.

(12) MacIver K, Lloyd DM, Kelly S, Roberts N, Nurmikko T. Phantom limb pain, cortical reorganization and the therapeutic effect of mental imagery. *Brain* 2008;131:2181–2191.

(13) Ypsilantis E, Tang TY. Pre-emptive analgesia for chronic limb pain after amputation for peripheral vascular disease: a systematic review. *Ann Vasc Surg* 2010;24:1139–1146.

(14) Karanikolas M, Aretha D, Tsolakis I, et al. Optimized perioperative analgesia reduces chronic phantom limb pain intensity, prevalence, and frequency: a prospective, randomized, clinical trial. *Anesthesiology* 2011;114:1144–1154.

(15) Borghi B, D'Addabbo M, White PF, et al. The use of prolonged peripheral neural blockade after lower extremity amputation: the effect on symptoms associated with phantom limb syndrome. *Anesth Analg* 2010;111:1308–1315.

(16) Rathmell JP, Kehlet H. Do we have the tools to prevent phantom limb pain? *Anesthesiology* 2011;114:1021–1024.

(17) Mulvey MR, Bagnall AM, Johnson MI, Marchant PR. Transcutaneous electrical nerve stimulation (TENS) for phantom pain and stump pain following amputation in adults. *Cochrane Database Syst Rev* 2010:CD007264.

(18) Ramachandran VS, Altschuler EL. The use of visual feedback, in particular mirror visual feedback, in restoring brain function. *Brain* 2009;132:1693–1710.

(19) Chan BL, Witt R, Charrow AP, et al. Mirror therapy for phantom limb pain. *N Engl J Med* 2007;357:2206–2207.

(20) Bittar RG, Otero S, Carter H, Aziz TZ. Deep brain stimulation for phantom limb pain. *J Clin Neurosci* 2005;12:399–404.

(21) Viswanathan A, Phan PC, Burton AW. Use of spinal cord stimulation in the treatment of phantom limb pain: case series and review of the literature. *Pain Pract* 2010;10:479–484.

(22) Ewalt JR, Randall GC, Morris H. The phantom limb. *Psychosom Med* 1947;9:118–123.

(23) Henderson WR, Smyth GE. Phantom limbs. *J Neurol Neurosurg Psychiatry* 1948;11:88–112.

(24) Abramson AS, Feibel A. The phantom phenomenon: its use and disuse. *Bull N Y Acad Med* 1981;57:99–112.

(25) Sherman RA, Sherman CJ. Prevalence and characteristics of chronic phantom limb pain among American veterans. Results of a trial survey. *Am J Phys Med* 1983;62:227–238.

(26) Sherman RA, Sherman CJ, Parker L. Chronic phantom and stump pain among American veterans: results of a survey. *Pain* 1984;18:83–95.

(27) Pohjolainen T. A clinical evaluation of stumps in lower limb amputees. *Prosthet Orthot Int* 1991;15:178–184.

(28) Wartan SW, Hamann W, Wedley JR, McColl I. Phantom pain and sensation among British veteran amputees. *Br J Anaesth* 1997;78:652–659.

(29) Kooijman CM, Dijkstra PU, Geertzen JH, Elzinga A, van der Schans CP. Phantom pain and phantom sensations in upper limb amputees: an epidemiological study. *Pain* 2000;87:33–41.

(30) Ephraim PL, Wegener ST, MacKenzie EJ, Dillingham TR, Pezzin LE. Phantom pain, residual limb pain, and back pain in amputees: results of a national survey. *Arch Phys Med Rehabil* 2005;86:1910–1919.

(31) Taghipour H, Moharamzad Y, Mafi AR, et al. Quality of life among veterans with war-related unilateral lower extremity amputation: a long-term survey in a prosthesis center in Iran. *J Orthop Trauma* 2009;23:525–530.

(32) Kern U, Busch V, Rockland M, Kohl M, Birklein F. [Prevalence and risk factors of phantom limb pain and phantom limb sensations in Germany. A nationwide field survey]. *Schmerz* 2009;23:479–488.

(33) Lotze M, Flor H, Grodd W, Larbig W, Birbaumer N. Phantom movements and pain. An fMRI study in upper limb amputees. *Brain* 2001;124:2268–2277.

Chapter 21

Pain in Parkinson's disease

Patients with Parkinson's disease (PD) predominantly suffer from motor disturbances. These patients however, may also be afflicted with several non-motor symptoms, including pain. The non-motor symptoms are common, occur in all stages of PD, and are probably under-reported and under-treated (1). Because pain is a key determinant of quality of life, pain in PD should be recognized, appropriately classified, and treated.

Clinical case vignette

A 59-year-old male schoolteacher with a history of arterial hypertension presented with pain in his right leg which had started 3 years ago. The pain was located in the right thigh, and from there it radiated down to the lower leg and also up to the lumbar spinal region. The pain was constant and was aggravated by standing for several hours or after vigorous walking. The patient felt increasingly challenged, because as a schoolteacher, he spent most of his time standing in front of his class. His general practitioner first referred him to an orthopedic surgeon who ordered an MRI scan of the lumbar spinal cord. Spondylosis of several lumbar segments was diagnosed. A non-steroidal anti-inflammatory drug (NSAID) was prescribed and the patient was administered several courses of physical therapy. The therapist emphasized strengthening of the spinal muscles and for a time, the patient experienced some pain relief. When the pain recurred, the patient consulted a second orthopedic surgeon who performed anesthetic blocks of several lumbar roots with lidocaine. The patient observed no effect and the pain intensified. Approximately 1 year after the onset of the pain, the patient additionally observed some numbness in the right leg. He was referred to a neurologist who considered the differential diagnoses of left hemisphere lesion of the brain such as a stroke or tumor, of a lumbar radicular lesion, and of polyneuropathy of the mononeuritis multiplex type. An MRI

scan of the brain showed mild periventricular white matter lesions, compatible with a history of arterial hypertension, but no other abnormalities. A spinal MRI scan confirmed no new findings when compared with a scan taken the previous year. A neurophysiological examination was performed. Somatosensory evoked potentials with stimulation of the tibial nerve were normal, excluding major conduction failure of the spinal cord. Nerve conduction studies of the sural and tibial nerves on both sides showed mild reductions in amplitudes and normal conduction velocities. A peripheral neuropathy was diagnosed and laboratory tests to clarify the etiology of the neuropathy were ordered. Serum chemistry, complete blood count, erythrocyte sedimentation rate, serum vitamin B12 concentration, serum protein electrophoresis, antinuclear antibodies, and a glucose tolerance test were all normal. A diagnosis of "asymmetric idiopathic painful peripheral neuropathy" was made. Because the clinical and electrophysiological findings were only mildly abnormal, the neurologist opted against more invasive tests (i.e., lumbar puncture and sural nerve biopsy) and prescribed symptomatic treatment with pregabalin 75 mg bid. The patient experienced some relief, downgrading his pain intensity from 5 to 3 on a numeric rating scale (NRS) of 0–10. He remained satisfied with this regimen until 6 months later when his ambulation was further impaired by a feeling of stiffness in the right leg. He started using a walking stick and sensed that he was dragging his right leg. There were occasional falls due to tripping over the right foot. When the patient consulted the neurologist again, a rigid–akinetic syndrome involving the right side of the body was noted on examination. His handwriting displayed micrography. When walking, he displayed a slightly stooped posture, short shuffling steps, and a reduced arm swing on the right. Upon passive movement of the arms, mild rigidity accentuated on the right side was evident. A diagnosis of Parkinson's disease (PD) was made, and the patient received a combination of levodopa/benserazide and a dopamine agonist. When the patient was seen again 4 weeks later, the motor symptoms had markedly improved and the leg pain had diminished in intensity to 2/10.

Discussion

The recent attention to non-motor symptoms in PD (1, 2) is attributable to two factors. Together, motor and non-motor symptoms significantly impact quality of life and must be addressed (3). Non-motor symptoms in isolation may also be indicative of a presymptomatic or pre-motor stage in PD. Reduction in the sense of smell, rapid eye movement disorder, constipation, and depression are recognized pre-motor symptoms while apathy, fatigue, and pain are considered possible pre-motor symptoms (2).

Pain in PD may occur in the early stages of the disease. With other signs and symptoms yet subtle, the presence of pain in isolation may be misleading and result in a delayed diagnosis. In a report of a 65-year-old patient with arm pain for 2 years, PD was finally diagnosed with the development of tremor in her right leg (4). Yet another case presented in the literature involved a patient who presented with leg pain, as in this vignette. Securing a diagnosis was further complicated by the young age of the patient (5). A final consideration is that PD tends to impact the upper limbs first, and a presentation with lower limb symptoms may be unexpected, resulting in inappropriate diagnostic procedures.

Non-motor symptoms may be present throughout the course of PD, and pain is a major component of the non-motor symptom complex. In three prevalence studies, pain was present in 21 to 46% of PD patients (2). The results of a French cross-sectional study found prevalence as high as 62% (6); pain had an average 60 mm of 100 mm on a visual analog scale, twice that of control patients.

Pain in PD is classified according to six distinct categories: 1. a musculoskeletal problem related to poor posture, awkward mechanical function, or physical wear and tear; 2. PD-related central or visceral pain; 3. pain due to fluctuations (dyskinesia and dystonia pain, pain in off-periods); 4. nocturnal pain (linked to restless legs, to nocturnal akinesia); 5. orofacial pain; 6. peripheral limb pain due to edema or limb pain that is drug-induced (2).

Direct PD-associated pain and secondary pain due to the sequelae of PD are also differentiated (1). For example, central pain is regarded as a direct consequence of the neurotransmitter disequilibrium of PD. Dyskinesia-related pain is also regarded as direct PD-associated pain. In contrast, a musculoskeletal problem due to poor posture is classified as secondary. Orofacial pain, caused by bruxism, is considered secondary, but because of its potential response to dopaminergic treatment it may also be directly linked to PD.

Pain in Parkinson's disease

Dopamine can modulate pain at several levels within the nervous system, including the spinal cord, thalamus, periaqueductal grey area, basal ganglia, and cingulate cortex (1). The cortical–basal ganglia–thalamic circuit is involved in modulating the motor, emotional, autonomic, and cognitive responses to pain (7). Several findings point to abnormal pain processing in PD patients. For example, PD patients with central pain had lower heat pain and laser pinprick thresholds, higher laser-evoked potential (LEP) amplitudes, and less habituation of sympathetic sudomotor responses to repetitive pain stimuli than PD patients without pain and control subjects. Furthermore, these responses were significantly attenuated after the administration of levodopa (8). A possible explanation for this occurrence is the dysfunction of dopamine-dependent autonomic centers which regulate autonomic function and inhibitory control of pain. Other studies found lower thresholds to heat pain on the involved side of PD patients (9).

In one study involving six patients with nocturnal pain and restless legs syndrome, there was marked improvement of pain after overnight apomorphine infusion (10). Also, the use of deep brain stimulation of the subthalamic nucleus and bilateral pallidal stimulation improved pain during levodopa off-periods (11, 12). Finally, patients given subthalamic stimulation believed that their pain had subsided even if other types of pain, mostly musculoskeletal, were induced by the treatment itself (13).

Imaging studies also support the concept of abnormal pain processing in this disease. PD patients in the off state had increased pain-induced cortical activation in a PET study; conversely, cortical activation was reduced during the on state (14). Of interest, this was not altered by apomorphine, a strong stimulator of the dopaminergic system (15). Manipulations of the pallidum, either surgically or by electrical stimulation, have alleviated pain in PD patients, indicating a role of this structure in pain modulation (7). Muscular pain is also thought to involve central as well as peripheral mechanisms (16). Impulses from the peripheral nervous system may also be influential. Skin biopsy analyses show loss of intraepidermal nerve fibers (17), and a disproportionally high percentage of PD patients have peripheral neuropathy; the use of levodopa is associated with polyneuropathy linked to B12 deficiency (18, 19).

A significant association between pain and depression scores is evident in PD patients. This association, together with the inconstant response of pain symptoms to dopaminergic drugs, gives credence to the concept that serotonin and norepinephrin, play a role in pain in PD patients. Indeed, the selective serotonin and norepinephrine reuptake inhibitor duloxetine improved pain in a small study that examined PD patients (20).

Most authors suggest a multidisciplinary approach (7). Physical therapy is warranted to maintain mobility and to prevent contractures. Conventional analgesics like NSAIDs may provide some symptomatic relief if pain is due to comorbid rheumatologic and orthopedic complications. Dopaminergic treatment may help to improve musculoskeletal pain by reducing akinesia and rigidity. The effect of dopaminergic agents on pain however, remains controversial because studies have yielded conflicting results (7). An analgesic antidepressant may be prescribed as described above. Deep brain stimulation of the subthalamic nucleus and globus pallidus, as with dopaminergic therapy, appears to provide some pain relief. This is confirmed by some studies but not in others (13, 21, 22).

References

(1) Chaudhuri KR, Schapira AH. Non-motor symptoms of Parkinson's disease: dopaminergic pathophysiology and treatment. *Lancet Neurol* 2009;8:464–474.

(2) Chaudhuri KR, Odin P, Antonini A, Martinez-Martin P. Parkinson's disease: the non-motor issues. *Parkinsonism Relat Disord* 2011;17:717–723.

(3) Martinez-Martin P, Rodriguez-Blazquez C, Kurtis MM, Chaudhuri KR. The impact of non-motor symptoms on health-related quality of life of patients with Parkinson's disease. *Mov Disord* 2011;26:399–406.

(4) Gilbert GJ. Biceps pain as the presenting symptom of Parkinson disease: effective treatment with L-dopa. *South Med J* 2004;97:776–777.

(5) Sekeff-Sallem FA, Barbosa ER. Diagnostic pitfalls in Parkinson's disease: case report. *Arq Neuropsiquiatr* 2007;65:348–351.

(6) Negre-Pages L, Regragui W, Bouhassira D, Grandjean H, Rascol O. Chronic pain in Parkinson's disease: the cross-sectional French DoPaMiP survey. *Mov Disord* 2008;23:1361–1369.

(7) Ha AD, Jankovic J. Pain in Parkinson's disease. *Mov Disord* 2012;**27**:485–491.

(8) Schestatsky P, Kumru H, Valls-Sole J, et al. Neurophysiologic study of central pain in patients with Parkinson disease. *Neurology* 2007;69: 2162–2169.

(9) Djaldetti R, Shifrin A, Rogowski Z, Sprecher E, Melamed E, Yarnitsky D. Quantitative measurement of pain sensation in patients with Parkinson disease. *Neurology* 2004;62:2171–2175.

(10) Reuter I, Ellis CM, Ray Chaudhuri K. Nocturnal subcutaneous apomorphine infusion in Parkinson's disease and restless legs syndrome. *Acta Neurol Scand* 1999;100:163–167.

(11) Loher TJ, Burgunder JM, Weber S, Sommerhalder R, Krauss JK. Effect of chronic pallidal deep brain stimulation on off period dystonia and sensory symptoms in advanced Parkinson's disease. *J Neurol Neurosurg Psychiatry* 2002;73:395–399.

(12) Witjas T, Kaphan E, Regis J, et al. Effects of chronic subthalamic stimulation on nonmotor fluctuations in Parkinson's disease. *Mov Disord* 2007;22:1729–1734.

(13) Kim HJ, Jeon BS, Lee JY, Paek SH, Kim DG. The benefit of subthalamic deep brain stimulation on pain in Parkinson disease: a 2-year follow-up study. *Neurosurgery* 2011;70:18–23.

(14) Brefel-Courbon C, Payoux P, Thalamas C, et al. Effect of levodopa on pain threshold in Parkinson's disease: a clinical and positron emission tomography study. *Mov Disord* 2005;20:1557–1563.

(15) Dellapina E, Gerdelat-Mas A, Ory-Magne F, et al. Apomorphine effect on pain threshold in Parkinson's disease: a clinical and positron emission tomography study. *Mov Disord* 2011;26:153–157.

(16) Tinazzi M, Recchia S, Simonetto S, et al. Muscular pain in Parkinson's disease and nociceptive processing assessed with CO_2 laser-evoked potentials. *Mov Disord* 2010;25:213–220.

(17) Nolano M, Provitera V, Estraneo A, et al. Sensory deficit in Parkinson's disease: evidence of a cutaneous denervation. *Brain* 2008;131:1903–1911.

(18) Rajabally YA, Martey J. Neuropathy in Parkinson disease: Prevalence and determinants. *Neurology* 2011;77:1947–1950.

(19) Toth C, Breithaupt K, Ge S, et al. Levodopa, methylmalonic acid, and neuropathy in idiopathic Parkinson disease. *Ann Neurol* 2010;68:28–36.

(20) Djaldetti R, Yust-Katz S, Kolianov V, Melamed E, Dabby R. The effect of duloxetine on primary pain symptoms in Parkinson disease. *Clin Neuropharmacol* 2007;30:201–205.

(21) Kim HJ, Jeon BS, Paek SH. Effect of deep brain stimulation on pain in Parkinson disease. *J Neurol Sci* 2011;310:251–255.

(22) Maruo T, Saitoh Y, Hosomi K, et al. Deep brain stimulation of the subthalamic nucleus improves temperature sensation in patients with Parkinson's disease. *Pain* 2011;152:860–865.

Chapter 22

Pain associated with amyotrophic lateral sclerosis (ALS)

Pain can be associated with neurological conditions not normally linked to damage or disruption of specific pain or sensory pathways. Whether these forms of pain should be described as "neuropathic" is debatable, yet they are prominent problems faced by patients. The loss of normal muscle control in a patient with a motor disorder, such as progressive ALS, can generate several forms of pain because of impaired limb and spine architecture and the inability to move limbs promptly when they are poorly aligned. In conditions with disease of lower motor neurons, abnormal cramp discharges can also arise.

Clinical case vignette

A 54-year-old right-handed man developed slurring of speech followed by difficulty swallowing and walking over a 1-year period. Dysphagia was noted for solids, liquids, and tablets. Although he had previously run up to 10 km daily, his walking became slow and difficult and he could barely complete 2 km. He noted weakness and wasting of his calf muscles and generalized muscle twitching. He denied sensory, sphincter, or cognitive problems. Hyperlipidemia, psoriasis, hepatitis as a child, and a benign neck lymph node biopsy were features of his previous medical history. His medications included numerous vitamins and supplements, long-acting niacin for hyperlipidemia, and aspirin. His father had died of ALS at age 61.

Neurological examination identified dysarthria. He had tongue fasciculations but no definite tongue atrophy or weakness, and otherwise normal cranial nerves. He had spasticity of his arms and legs, scattered limb muscle fasciculations, and weakness of intrinsic hand muscles, ankle dorsiflexors, and ankle plantar flexors. There was atrophy in his hand muscles. He had brisk deep tendon reflexes (+3/4) throughout, a jaw jerk, Hoffman signs, and downgoing plantar responses. Sensory examination was normal. His gait was slowed and spastic. He was prescribed riluzole.

By 2 years after the onset of his neurological symptoms, the patient was anarthric, had developed more extensive wasting, and had more severe weakness of both his hands and legs. He had severe dysphagia with secondary weight loss and there was a fall in his vital capacity to 61% of the predicted value (112% 5 months earlier). He declined a percutaneous gastroscopy tube for enteral feeding.

Electrophysiological studies identified low amplitude lower limb motor CMAPs without dispersion, block or conduction slowing. Sensory potentials were normal. Needle electromyography identified fibrillations and positive sharp waves in the following muscles: left first dorsal interosseous, left deltoid, left and right tibialis anterior, left gastrocnemius, left vastus medialis, right abductor pollicus brevis, C6 and L5 paraspinal muscles, and the tongue.

Normal (negative) laboratory studies included: genetic analysis for SOD1 mutation, genetic analysis for androgen receptor triplet (Kennedy's disease), complete blood count, ESR, electrolytes, urea, creatinine, calcium, aluminum, ferritin, iron, TIBC, lipid profile (borderline elevated cholesterol), TSH, B12, SPEP (serum protein electrophoresis), ALT, GGT, AST, ANA, RF, glucose, urinalysis, HIV 1 and 2 serology, syphilis serology, AchR antibody, urinary copper excretion, ceruloplasmin, CT chest, abdomen and pelvis, MR brain, thoracic spine, and lumbar spine. Creatine kinase was elevated at 833 (normal, <195 U/L). MRI of C spine showed multilevel degenerative changes with mild cervical spinal stenosis.

Pain description

At 2 years following the onset of his ALS symptoms, the patient noted painful cramps and spasms in his hands and forearms, sometimes related to position. He had experienced similar intermittent symptoms over the past 2 years but they became more prominent later as he developed severe weakness of his hands. Although he also described fasciculations, he did not categorize them as painful. Earlier in his course, he also described painful tingling sensations radiating from his neck down into his arms, a symptom suggestive of Lhermitte's phenomenon. These issues prompted his investigation with cervical spine MR imaging; the degenerative changes identified however did not account for the progressive weakness and atrophy involving all of his limbs.

Discussion

This patient presented with classical symptoms and signs of bulbar and limb amyotrophic lateral sclerosis (ALS). His first symptoms were dysarthria and dysphagia, then limb spasticity and weakness. Electrophysiological studies confirmed widespread limb (and tongue) denervation indicating lower motor neuron dropout. Other investigations failed to identify an alternative explanation for his severe, progressive course. As his condition progressed, he developed new symptoms that included pain and cramping in the hands. The pain did not have typical descriptive qualities of neuropathic pain because there was an absence of burning, tingling, or electrical sensations. Earlier shooting sensations of pain may have been due to concurrent cervical spinal degenerative disc disease.

Pain in ALS

Although ALS primarily targets motor units, patients with this disorder can experience pain (1). As is apparent from this case description, symptoms of pain in ALS typically differ from neuropathic pain symptoms such as burning, electrical, tingling, prickling, and hypersensitivity that are associated with disease of the sensory system. Rather the patient noted cramping and spasms. Diseased motor units in ALS develop spontaneous activity that accounts for both fasciculations as well as painful cramping of major muscle groups. The molecular trigger for this activity is not fully understood.

Another important quality of pain experienced by patients with ALS is an exaggeration of pre-ALS musculoskeletal damage. This patient also presented with a pre-existing cervical spondylosis and as early muscle weakness developed, he developed radicular-like shooting discomfort. Patients with paralysis from ALS have difficulty moving limbs that are placed in awkward and uncomfortable positions. Because most patients have intact sensation, their failure to protect

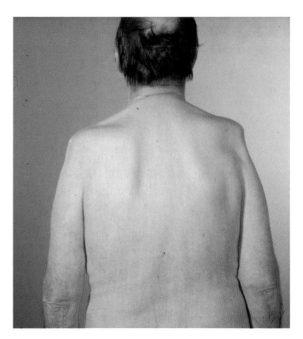

Figure 22.1 Wasted shoulder girdle muscles in a patient (not the patient in this vignette) with ALS. Note the loss of deltoid muscle on the right and of the supraspinatus muscle on the left. Weakness of axial muscles with loss of their normal supportive function may contribute toward musculoskeletal pain in ALS patients.

their limbs from injury can account for pain. Falls may be frequent in patients with footdrop or limb spasticity from ALS. Spinal pain can be especially problematic in patients that cannot adjust their position in beds or wheelchairs. There may be denervation of truncal spinal muscles that maintain proper alignment of the neck and lower back [Figure 22.1]. Finally, spasticity may be severe in patients with more upper motor neuron involvement. Patients with primary lateral sclerosis, a cousin of ALS, can have very prominent and painful spasticity.

The prevalence of pain in ALS has had limited attention. Chio et al. (2) reported pain in 56.9% of 160 patients, a higher prevalence than in controls (33.1%). The patients had ALS for a mean of 31 months and described their pain as largely involving the extremities. There were no significant differences in the frequency of pain in relationship with the type of ALS onset. Pain increased in frequency and intensity with progression of the disease and interfered with activities of daily living. In a separate study, 19% of ALS patients rated pain as 4 or greater on a six-point scale. Pain correlated with feelings of hopelessness, suffering, and depression (3).

Treatment of pain from ALS may include simple measures such as repositioning, appropriate padding, and physiotherapy of impaired limbs. Patients may require neck support, particularly when in a wheelchair. Cramps may be treated with levetiracetam, physiotherapy, physical exercise, or hydrotherapy (see the recent EFNS guideline on the clinical management of ALS (4)). Painful spasticity may be treated with baclofen, dantrolene, tizanidine, or botulinum toxin injections. Simple analgesics or low-dose opioid preparations may be used in ALS patients, although respiratory depression and constipation are difficult side-effects in advanced disease. The author has noted some anecdotal benefit from the use of gabapentin or pregabalin.

References

(1) Wicks P. Reassessing received wisdom in ALS–pain is common when studied systematically. *Eur J Neurol* 2012;19:531–532.

(2) Chiò A, Canosa A, Gallo S, et al. Pain in amyotrophic lateral sclerosis: a population-based controlled study. *Eur J Neurol* 2012;19:551–555.

(3) Ganzini L, Johnston WS, Hoffman WF. Correlates of suffering in amyotrophic lateral sclerosis. *Neurology* 1999;52:1434–1440.

(4) Andersen PM, Abrahams S, Borasio GD, et al. EFNS guidelines on the Clinical Management of Amyotrophic Lateral Sclerosis (MALS) – revised report of an EFNS task force. *Eur J Neurol* 2012;19:360–375.

Pain in Brown-Séquard syndrome

Brown-Séquard syndrome is classically encountered in acute traumatic spine injuries with hemisection of the spinal cord. Rarely, it can also be encountered in cervical spondylosis. This vignette illustrates central pain of spinal origin in a patient with cervical myelopathy and incomplete Brown-Séquard syndrome.

Clinical case vignette

A 61-year-old man with a history of cervical pain attributed to spondylosis had an acute episode of pain radiating into the right arm with numbness of the 3rd to 5th fingers. Spinal MRI confirmed degenerative spondylosis without root compression. Cerebrospinal fluid analyzed after lumbar tap, to exclude infectious radiculitis, was normal. After symptomatic treatment with NSAIDs and muscle relaxants over 5 days, the symptoms resolved. During the week after discharge from hospital, the patient developed burning pain and loss of temperature sense of the right half of his body. He noticed the loss of temperature sensation when the use of heat pads for pain relief resulted in burns to the skin. The face and neck were not involved. The patient was readmitted to hospital. On examination, a mild central hemiparesis on the left, reduction of vibration and position sense on the left, and loss of pain and temperature sense on the right were observed below C3. A second spinal MRI confirmed a lesion at the level of C3 on T2-weighted images with a ventrolateral accentuation [Figure 23.1]. Cerebrospinal fluid was again normal, and spinal ischemia, possibly related to spinal stenosis, was diagnosed. The patient was started on secondary prevention of ischemic events with ASA 100 mg, and gabapentin, 600 mg tid, was administered for central pain. This led to a moderate reduction of the pain for the first 6 weeks although the effect abated from this time onward. One year later, the patient's symptoms still had not improved and he was seen for a second opinion. An incomplete Brown-Séquard syn-

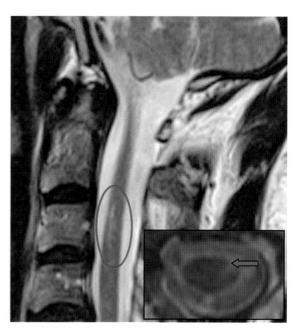

Figure 23.1. T2-weighted spinal MRI of the patient. A left ventrolateral lesion is visible at the level of C3 (oval). The inset shows the lesion at the horizontal plane (arrow). Courtesy of Prof. Solymosi, Department of Neuroradiology, University Hospital of Würzburg.

drome was present on examination. Very mild hemiparesis on the left was manifested by reduced strength of finger extension and abnormal one-legged hopping. Sensory findings were as described above, and the dissociation of sensory modalities was confirmed by quantitative sensory testing [Figure 23.2]. The patient's pain drawing is shown in Figure 23.3. Neurophysiological studies revealed pathological magnetic evoked potentials recorded from the right lower leg, but normal somatosensory evoked potentials when stimulating the tibial nerve. The lesion on T2-weighted MRI was smaller in size than previously assessed. The gabapentin was changed to pregabalin 150 mg tid, which reduced the pain intensity to 3/10 with fluctuations.

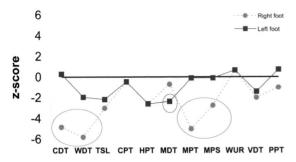

Figure 23.2. Quantitative sensory testing of the dorsal foot revealed increased temperature perception thresholds and loss of pain perception (red circles) at the contralateral side and an ipsilateral increase in tactile detection thresholds (blue circle) compared with controls (black line). Calculation according to (7). CDT: cold detection threshold; WDT: warm detection threshold; TSL: thermal sensory limen (ability to detect temperature differences); CPT: cold pain threshold; HPT: heat pain threshold; MDT; mechanical pain detection threshold; MPT: mechanical pain threshold; MPS: mechanical pain sensitivity; WUR: wind-up ratio of ten painful stimuli; VDT: vibration detection threshold; PPT: pressure pain threshold.

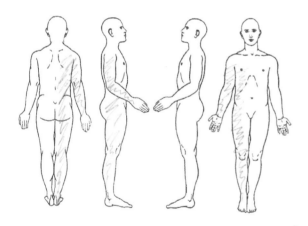

Fig. 23.3. Pain drawing as depicted by the patient. Note sparing of face and upper cervical segments.

Pain description

The patient's pain was described as burning with a maximal intensity of 8/10 and a mean intensity of 5/10. The patient could not identify aggravating factors, but there were spontaneous fluctuations. Warming alleviated the pain but had to be used with care because of the risk of burns. The patient admitted to suicidal ideation when the pain was intense. Standard analgesics had no effect.

Discussion

Brown-Séquard syndrome was first described in 1850 by the neurologist Dr. Charles Edouard Brown-Séquard. Brown-Séquard syndrome is defined as an ipsilateral loss of motor function and proprioception combined with contralateral loss of pain and temperature sensation due to spinothalamic tract dysfunction. The clinical picture reflects hemisection or hemicompression of the spinal cord with ipsilateral loss of function of the tracts crossing above the lesion (corticospinal tract, dorsal column), contralateral loss of function of the tract axons crossing below the level (spinothalamic tract), and only mild loss of function of such qualities that are represented in more than one tract, like epicritic sensation (dorsal column and spinothalamic tract). Herniated cervical discs or cervical spinal stenosis may also cause Brown-Séquard syndrome (1, 2). Pain may be part of this syndrome but is rarely described in detail. Pain as occurs in Brown-Séquard syndrome is comparable to other forms of spinal cord damage.

Pain in spinal cord injury

Central neuropathic pain is a well-known sequel of spinal cord injury. In a follow-up study of 100 patients, pain was present in 64% at 6 months after the injury, and 21% of these described it as severe (3). In spinal cord injury, pain has been well studied and described in several publications (for review see Siddall and Finnerup (4)), in contrast to Brown-Séquard syndrome. Patients with spinal cord injury pain suffer from various types of pain including musculoskeletal, at the injured cord level, and pain below the injured cord level. Aspects of "below level" pain are most related to the case described above. Patients describe a constant throbbing, burning, and stabbing pain that is diffusely located caudal to the level of the injury. The pain may be associated with hyperalgesia.

The pathophysiology of pain caused by a spinal cord lesion is assumed to include neuronal hyperexcitability, reduced inhibition, and neuronal reorganization or plasticity. Increased neuronal excitability may be the consequence of the dramatic increase in excitatory amino acids resulting from a major lesion of nervous structures. In addition, there is activation of glial cells, which in turn release pro-inflammatory cytokines and chemokines that act on neurons (5). An important mechanism is the probable loss of descending and local inhibition. Damage to the ascending and descending pathways in the spinal cord results in disruption of local inhibitory interneurons and loss or decreased influence of supraspinal and propriospinal inhibitory pathways. Recently, spinal and supraspinal reorganization have been linked to spinal cord injury pain. For example, diffusion tensor imaging showed anatomical changes in pain-related regions as well as regions of the classic reward circuitry, specifically the nucleus accumbens and orbitofrontal, dorsolateral prefrontal, and posterior parietal cortex (6).

References

(1) Sani S, Boco T, Deutsch H. Cervical stenosis presenting with acute Brown-Sequard syndrome: case report. *Spine (Phila Pa 1976)* 2005;30:E481–E483.

(2) Sayer FT, Vitali AM, Low HL, Paquette S, Honey CR. Brown-Sequard syndrome produced by C3-C4 cervical disc herniation: a case report and review of the literature. *Spine (Phila Pa 1976)* 2008;33: E279–E282.

(3) Siddall PJ, McClelland JM, Rutkowski SB, Cousins MJ. A longitudinal study of the prevalence and characteristics of pain in the first 5 years following spinal cord injury. *Pain* 2003;103:249–257.

(4) Siddall PJ, Finnerup NB. Chapter 46 Pain following spinal cord injury. *Handb Clin Neurol* 2006;81:689–703.

(5) McMahon SB, Malcangio M. Current challenges in glia-pain biology. *Neuron* 2009;64:46–54.

(6) Gustin SM, Wrigley PJ, Siddall PJ, Henderson LA. Brain anatomy changes associated with persistent neuropathic pain following spinal cord injury. *Cereb Cortex* 2010;20:1409–1419.

(7) Rolke R, Baron R, Maier C, et al. Quantitative sensory testing in the German Research Network on Neuropathic Pain (DFNS): standardized protocol and reference values. *Pain* 2006;123:231–243.

Pain in syringomyelia

Syringomyelia is a disorder in which a cavity forms within the spinal cord, leading to a specific combination of symptoms. Some authors use the term syringomyelia exclusively for cavities outside of the central canal, and hydromyelia for cavities that develop from central canal dilatation lined with ependymal cells. This chapter uses the term syringomyelia for both conditions.

Clinical case vignette

A 23-year-old male experienced a severe accident while hiking in the mountains. He had polytrauma, including a brain contusion and multiple bone fractures. Hospitalized for several months, he recovered well, leading a normal professional and private life until the age of 70. He then presented with a 9-month history of pain and paresthesiae in his right hand. Six months prior, he had also noted weakness of the right hand. His walking ability had declined. Having no previous impairments, he became exhausted after 1 h of walking at a normal pace. In particular, his left leg grew tired and needed to be pulled along. He denied having any relevant pain or weakness until 3 years prior when he noticed mild, intermittent pain and paresthesiae in the left lower arm, including the entire hand.

On examination, the patient was fully conscious and cooperative. His gait was ataxic and tandem gait was not possible. One-legged hopping was normal on the right, but impaired on the left. There was mild muscle atrophy of the left arm and leg muscles, more pronounced than on the right. He had bilateral weakness and wasting of the intrinsic hand muscles. Tendon jerks were present and brisker on the left. The Babinski sign was present bilaterally. Sensory testing revealed loss of sensation for touch, pinprick, and loss of temperature sense on the left below the level of T4 and reduced pain and temperature of the right arm [Figure 24.1]. There was loss of vibration perception at the right malleolus but normal on the

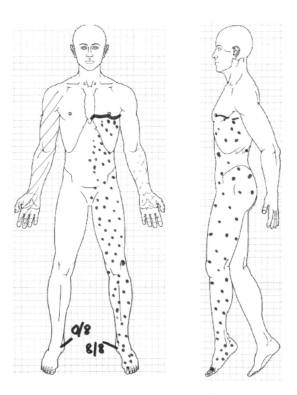

Figure 24.1. Sketch depicting patient's sensory loss.

left side. Laboratory tests were unremarkable. EMG studies revealed fibrillations from the left first dorsal interosseus muscle, mild prolongation of somatosensory evoked potentials from the tibial nerve, and normal motor and sensory nerve conduction studies of the ulnar and median nerves on both sides. Amplitudes of magnetic evoked potentials were reduced after left cortical stimulation, with normal latencies. Spinal MRI showed an extensive cavity in the upper spinal cord that ranged from the 2nd cervical to the 2nd thoracic vertebral body [Figure 24.2]. Finally, degenerative spondylosis with segmental spinal stenosis accentuated at C3/4 to C4/5 was identified.

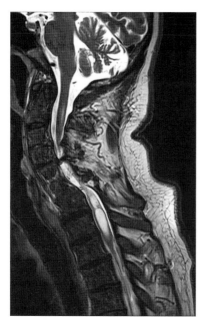
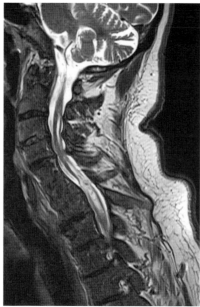
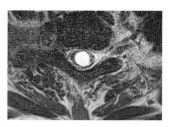
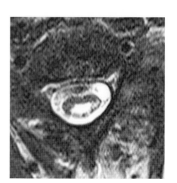

Figure 24.2. T2-weighted spinal MRI of the patient: (left and middle) sagittal, (right, upper and lower) axial reconstruction. Note the extended syrinx, spanning over more than seven segments (a). At its widest diameter at the level of Th 1/2, the syrinx has more than doubled the diameter of the cord and the remaining myelin is compressed. Courtesy of Prof. Solymosi, Department of Neuroradiology, University Hospital of Würzburg.

The patient consulted with a neurosurgeon but decided against surgical intervention. Pain treatment was initiated with pregabalin, which provided benefit.

Pain description

The patient described his pain in the right arm as alternating in quality: burning, aching, and pressing. He had intermittent electric-shock–like pain radiating into the right hand. Allodynia was absent although the patient reported a tingling sensation that was essentially continuous (paresthesiae) in the right arm. Generally, the pain in the left arm was milder, intermittent, and although present for several years, it had not motivated the patient to see a doctor. In addition to spontaneous fluctuations, there were also changes in pain intensity evoked by certain factors. Coughing, straining, bodily exertion, as well as psychological stress aggravated his symptoms.

Discussion

The term syringomyelia is ascribed to d'Angers in 1824 (1). The cystic cavity is typically found in the cervical spinal cord; if it extends upward into the medulla oblongata, the condition is called syringobulbia. There

are also cases of syringomyelia in the lumbar region. Most cases of syringomyelia are associated with developmental disorders, usually a Chiari I malformation. Acquired syringomyelia is thought to be caused by several factors. Trauma is likely the most common, the syrinx is then situated above the level of the spinal injury. A CSF leak after brachial plexus avulsion has also been described as a causative factor (2). Others include spinal arachnoiditis and spinal or infratentorial tumors.

Pain, segmental dissociated sensory loss, and atrophic paresis, generally of the hands, are typical clinical symptoms. The onset is usually insidious in both developmental and acquired cases. The quality and distribution of symptoms and signs are determined by the centromedullary localization of the lesion. This localization interrupts incoming lateral spinothalamic crossing tract fibers causing impairment of pain and temperature sensation bilaterally or ipsilateral to the paracentral extension of the syrinx (3) and thus leads to "dissociated" sensory loss. "Dissociated" refers to the selective involvement of pain and temperature sensibility with sparing of light touch, position, and vibration sensation. Quantitative sensory testing can aid in the diagnosis through detection of increased warm and cold thresholds and to a lesser degree, increased pain thresholds (4). Because the cervical cord is the most common localization, the ulnar border of the hand and forearm are often initially affected by dissociated sensory loss. In syringobulbia, the area may extend to the upper arm, the upper part of the chest and back and the face. The distribution may be uni- or bilateral. If the syrinx extends and involves the dorsal root entry zone, all sensory qualities are involved. Additional involvement may include anterior spinothalamic tracts, posterior columns, or corticospinal tracts. Loss of proprioceptive and tactile sensation may follow as well as increased vibration detection thresholds. Extension of the syrinx to the ventral horn induces wasting and weakness with fasciculations. The very large, irregular syrinx of the patient described above explains the combination of these symptoms. Thus, depending on the localization of the syrinx, there can be combined upper and lower motor signs in the arms or in the legs. There may be trophic changes in the hands including hyperkeratosis and edema. Horner's syndrome is frequently found (5). Syringobulbia may induce further cranial nerve symptoms including nystagmus, palatal weakness, and tongue atrophy with fasciculations (6).

Post-traumatic syringomyelia may manifest with symptoms in a time-frame anywhere from 3 months to 35 years after the trauma. Consequently, patients with a late motor and sensory deterioration or a newly developed pain syndrome after spinal cord injury should be evaluated for the presence of a post-traumatic syrinx. Typically, the patients develop an ascending sensory level, pain in the neck or arms, muscle weakness, and later spasticity. Syringomyelia symptoms develop in 1 to 9% of patients after spinal injury. Radiologically defined syringomyelia, in contrast, develops in up to 30% of spinal injury patients within 30 years after the injury (7). Traumatic syringomyelia is of the non-communicating variety without continuity to the fourth ventricle (3). The post-traumatic syrinx is usually localized next to the injury site and extends rostrally in 81%, caudally in 4%, and in both directions in 15% of cases. It may extend for more than ten vertebral levels (7).

The pathogenesis of post-traumatic syringomyelia is not entirely understood. Predisposing factors include increasing age, uncorrected kyphosis, cervical and thoracic level displaced fractures, and spinal instrumentation without decompression (8). There is an association with subarachnoid adhesions, spinal deformity, and stenosis. CSF flow in post-traumatic syringomyelia patients may be turbulent, and influenced by a locally tethered cord and blockage of the subarachnoid space by arachnoid scarring (7).

Pain in syringomyelia

Pain is a major complaint in a significant proportion of syringomyelia patients and is likely due to disordered neuronal processing in the damaged dorsal horn. Symptomatic syringomyelia is reported in only 1–9% of patients with spinal injury. Approximately 50% of patients with traumatic, and most patients with developmental syringomyelia suffer from pain. The pain quality in syringomyelia has been variously described as dull, aching, or burning (7). Paroxysmal shooting pain may also be present. Different types of pain may coexist in one patient (4). The pain is often perceived at or above the level of injury and may expand over time. Its intensity may be mild or severe. Constant or intermittent pain may occur. Coughing, sneezing, straining, or sitting can exacerbate the pain. Evoked pain is common, manifesting as allodynia or hyperalgesia (9). Some patients report persistent pain after evoked pain, i.e., after sensations or delayed sensations. Tingling and pins-and-needles sensations may also occur, as well as numbness.

Neuropathic arthropathy of the shoulder is another pain syndrome associated with post-traumatic syringomyelia (10). Neuropathic arthropathy is seen in 25% of patients with syringomyelia and occurs at the upper extremity in 80%. Patients present with shoulder pain, swelling of the shoulder or elbow, and decreased range of motion. Active forward flexion and abduction are most impaired, passive movements are painful. Loss of sensation in the shoulder area may be found. Diagnostic work-up includes radiographs of the shoulder which may show osteolysis of the humeral head and the glenoid process. The diagnosis of syringomyelia may be delayed if the patient initially presents for orthopedic evaluation. The pathophysiology of neuropathic arthropathy is assumed to include trophic disturbances due to lack of innervation and repetitive microtrauma because of reduced or lost pain sensation. Treatment consists in treating the underlying syrinx. Surgical manipulations at the shoulder alone may aggravate the situation, causing further deterioration (10). Pain in syringomyelia is classified as central neuropathic pain. The presence of thermal sensory deficits may be linked to the disinhibition theory of pain (11) and spinothalamic neurons are thought hyperexcitable. Alternatively, the thermosensory disinhibition theory proposes that central pain results from disruption of the normal inhibition of the pathways mediating thermal sensation in the nociceptive system (12).

There is no simple direct relationship between the magnitude of extent of sensory loss and the presence, quality, or intensity of neuropathic pain (9). In a recent study where 37 patients with syringomyelia were examined, the 27 patients with neuropathic pain were indistinguishable from those without pain in quantitative sensory testing, laser-evoked and somatosensory-evoked potentials, and three-dimensional MRI fiber tracking analyses (13). Among patients with neuropathic pain, those with greater structural damage as assessed by MR fractional anisotropy, had higher average daily pain intensity. This correlation was stronger in patients with spontaneous pain than in patients with both spontaneous and evoked pain. Patients with both spontaneous and evoked pain had less structural spinal cord damage and better preserved spinothalamic and lemniscal tract function. Pathophysiological mechanisms responsible for the various components of pain in syringomyelia are current topics of discussion (4). They also include supraspinal involvement.

Several surgical treatment options are available, including shunting of the syrinx to the subarachnoid space or to either the pleural or peritoneal cavities, spinal cord untethering with or without duraplasty, and cordectomy. An expert panel recently agreed that a surgical intervention is indicated in the setting of motor deterioration, but could not find sufficient evidence to recommend surgery in patients with asymptomatic syrinx or with sensory loss and pain as the only symptoms (14). There was no strong evidence to support the superiority of one surgical technique over the others, but some evidence appeared to confirm that spinal cord untethering with expansile duraplasty might be preferable. This method has not consistently benefitted patients although shunting and reducing the cyst volume in a large post-traumatic syrinx would seem to be a logical approach (14, 15). Arachnoidolysis, i.e., surgical loosening of arachnoid adhesion at the level of injury, seems to provide some benefit. It aims to restore normal CSF flow around the injured segment. In a small series of patients, the procedure led to reduction of cyst length in over 50% of cases as well as a decrease in pain (16). In a follow-up study that included 362 patients 12 years after surgery, approx-imately 10% of the patients had surgical procedures for progressively worsening neuropathic pain, their only symptom. In 47% of this group, surgery provided pain relief and enhanced quality of life (17). Finally, spinal cordectomy is a potential therapy for paraplegic patients with intractable symptoms. It offers reduced pain and improved quality of life in select patients (18).

References

(1) Nogues MA. Syringomyelia. In: Gilman, ed. *MedLink Neurology*. San Diego: MedLink Corporation.

(2) Scholsem M, Scholtes F, Belachew S, Martin D. Acquired tonsillar herniation and syringomyelia after pleural effusion aspiration: case report. *Neurosurgery* 2008;62:E1172–E1173; discussion E1173.

(3) Milhorat TH. Classification of syringomyelia. *Neurosurg Focus* 2000;8:E1.

(4) Attal N, Bouhassira D. Pain in syringomyelia/bulbia. *Handb Clin Neurol* 2006;81:705–713.

(5) Kerrison JB, Biousse V, Newman NJ. Isolated Horner's syndrome and syringomyelia. *J Neurol Neurosurg Psychiatry* 2000;69:131–132.

(6) Delpirou C, Heroum C, Blard JM, Pages M. [Acute onset syringomyelia: two cases]. *Rev Neurol (Paris)* 2001;157:692–694.

(7) Brodbelt AR, Stoodley MA. Post-traumatic syringomyelia: a review. *J Clin Neurosci* 2003;10: 401–408.

(8) Vannemreddy SS, Rowed DW, Bharatwal N. Posttraumatic syringomyelia: predisposing factors. *Br J Neurosurg* 2002;16:276–283.

(9) Ducreux D, Attal N, Parker F, Bouhassira D. Mechanisms of central neuropathic pain: a combined psychophysical and fMRI study in syringomyelia. *Brain* 2006;129:963–976.

(10) Atalar AC, Sungur M, Demirhan M, Ozger H. Neuropathic arthropathy of the shoulder associated with syringomyelia: a report of six cases. *Acta Orthop Traumatol Turc* 2010;44:328–336.

(11) Boivie J, Leijon G, Johansson I. Central post-stroke pain–a study of the mechanisms through analyses of the sensory abnormalities. *Pain* 1989;37:173–185.

(12) Craig AD, Chen K, Bandy D, Reiman EM. Thermosensory activation of insular cortex. *Nat Neurosci* 2000;3:184–190.

(13) Hatem SM, Attal N, Ducreux D, et al. Clinical, functional and structural determinants of central pain in syringomyelia. *Brain* 2010;133:3409–3422.

(14) Bonfield CM, Levi AD, Arnold PM, Okonkwo DO. Surgical management of post-traumatic

syringomyelia. *Spine (Phila Pa 1976)* 2010;35:S245–S258.

(15) Attal N, Parker F, Tadie M, Aghakani N, Bouhassira D. Effects of surgery on the sensory deficits of syringomyelia and predictors of outcome: a long term prospective study. *J Neurol Neurosurg Psychiatry* 2004;75:1025–1030.

(16) Aghakhani N, Baussart B, David P, et al. Surgical treatment of posttraumatic syringomyelia. *Neurosurgery* 2010;66:1120–1127; discussion 1127.

(17) Falci SP, Indeck C, Lammertse DP. Posttraumatic spinal cord tethering and syringomyelia: surgical treatment and long-term outcome. *J Neurosurg Spine* 2009;11:445–460.

(18) Gautschi OP, Seule MA, Cadosch D, et al. Health-related quality of life following spinal cordectomy for syringomyelia. *Acta Neurochir (Wien)* 2011;153:575–579.

Central pain with thalamic infarct

Although central pain can originate from diverse areas of the brain, lesions in the thalamus, in particular in its ventroposterior part, are particularly associated with chronic pain. Among the patients with post-stroke pain, approximately 60% have lesions in the thalamus (1). The importance of the ventroposterior part of the thalamus is illustrated in the vignette that follows.

Clinical case vignette

A 69-year-old right-handed woman presented with an 18-month history of pain in the right hand. She described the pain as continuous with an intensity of 7/10 and not aggravated by movement. The onset of the pain had been acute, accompanied by slight weakness of the right hand, and paresthesias of the right palm and the upper right lip. The patient had been investigated for carpal tunnel syndrome, and when this was negative, a CT head scan was performed which revealed a left thalamic infarct [Figure 25.1]. The patient had suffered from a right thalamic infarct 5 years earlier. This older infarct was also evident on the CT but the patient did not have residual deficits. A cardiac embolism likely was responsible for the lesions; the patient had received an aortic valve replacement 10 years earlier and was on anticoagulation. Concomitant disorders included arterial hypertension, compensated renal insufficiency, and reflux esophagitis. In addition to previous neurological examinations, medical, orthopedic, and rheumatological examinations had been performed which yielded no alternative causes of pain.

The patient described the pain in the right hand as deep and sore, like needles, but also numb. It was most intense on the palmar side of the first four fingers. Touch was perceived as unpleasant. Passive and active movement did not influence the pain. Cooling reduced the pain intensity which was 7/10 on most days.

Neurological examination revealed intact mental function and cranial nerves. Deep tendon reflexes were brisker on the right. Strength of finger adduction and abduction of the right hand was slightly reduced (4+/5 MRC grade). Grip strength with a medium-sized rubber bulb was 48 kPA on the left (normal) and 20 kPA on the right (reduced); otherwise motor power was normal. The finger–nose test was mildly dysmetric on the right, and rapid alternating movements of the right hand were slowed. Light touch of the palmar aspect of the fingers on the right was perceived as uncomfortable pins and needles (allodynia). The perception threshold for von Frey hairs was 4 mg on the left index finger, 28 mg on the right, indicating hypoesthesia. Moderate pressure was perceived as extremely painful, indicating hyperalgesia. Temperature and vibration sense were normal, and sensation was normal in the rest of the body.

The patient had seen several pain specialists and various pharmaceutical treatment regimens had been attempted. NSAIDs, flupirtine, and metamizole were without effect. Weak and strong opioids were used in low doses (e.g., oxycodone 10 mg), but were rapidly discontinued because of side-effects. Tricyclic antidepressants yielded the same results. Gabapentin was given at a dose of up to 1200 mg and in combination with desipramine. The patient only reported a maximal reduction of 1/10. Long-term side-effects included nausea, confusion, loss of appetite, constipation, headache, ankle edema, and itching. Therapeutic anticoagulation levels were rendered unstable by the above treatments.

At the time of consultation, the patient had discontinued all pain medication and was asking for new options. Pregabalin was started at a dose of 75 mg bid. Because the patient experienced an unstable gait and a sense of confusion, she discontinued the medication after 4 days. Physical therapy and cold water baths for the right hand were also prescribed. Three months later, she reported a moderate pain reduction to 6/10. The neurological findings were unchanged except for an increase in grip strength to 30 kPa on the right.

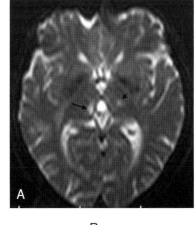

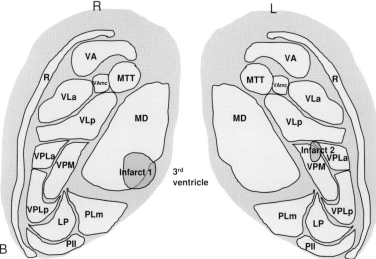

Figure 25.1 (A) Original MRI scan of the patient, showing a large thalamic infarct on the right (arrow) and a small thalamic infarct (arrowhead) on the left. Courtesy of Prof. Solymosi, Department of Neuroradiology, University Hospital of Würzburg. (B) Schematic diagram of the main thalamic nuclei (modified after Schmahmann (2)). The patient's infarcts are shown as dark structures. Nuclei involved in the patient's strokes: MD: mediodorsal nucleus; VPM: ventral posterior medial nucleus; VPL: ventral posterior medial lateral nucleus; a: anterior; p: posterior.

Discussion

Two aspects of this case history are significant: 1. the presence of bilateral thalamic infarcts, of which one led to central pain; 2. the patient's relative lack of response to pharmacological treatment.

The patient's first infarct occurred in the paramedian artery territory (2) [Figure 25.1Aa] which perfuses the posteromedial thalamus [Figure 25.1Bb]. These lesions usually lead to decreased level of consciousness, neuropsychologial disturbances, and abnormalities of vertical gaze. The patient did not remember any symptoms from the first stroke, likely because of her decreased level of consciousness at the time. The second stroke occurred in the territory of the inferolateral artery which supplies the ventrolateral thalamus including the ventral posterior lateral and medial nuclei. Infarcts in this area may lead to the classical features of thalamic syndrome that include sensory loss, impaired extremity movement and pain. Eighteen months after her stroke, our patient exhibited mild sensory loss and motor dysfunction but her pain remained severe.

The treatment of central neuropathic pain is difficult (3, 4). Randomized controlled trials are scarce, and although most give negative results, some progress has been made. Amitriptyline was of therapeutic benefit in a small trial (5). Lamotrigine showed a modest effect in one study (6). Success with gabapentin and pregabalin were reported in single case reports, but in a randomized controlled trial pregabalin did not result in more pain reduction than placebo (7). Opioids, in particular slow-release formulations like fentanyl patches, appear to benefit some patients (8). Given these limited results, stimulation procedures and ablative surgery have also been attempted. The latter had no effect on chronic pain (9). Deep brain stimulation, in particular of the periventricular grey regions and of the motor cortex, successfully alleviated pain in individual patients (10, 11).

Despite the high scores given on the NRS pain rating scale out of 10, our patient's distress was not severe enough to justify such treatment. Simpler physical measures proved adequate.

Central post-stroke pain

Chronic pain after stroke has been described in up to 55% of patients, but most of this pain is central and not directly linked to the cerebral ischemia (4). Pain after stroke may be associated with pre-existing chronic pain disorders. The most common chronic post-stroke pain that is indirectly related to the stroke is shoulder pain, which occurs in 30–40% of patients with stroke (4). It is related to sensory and motor deficits on the involved side, subluxation, and a limited range of movement.

In a population-based study in Denmark, the prevalence of definite or probable central post-stroke pain was 7.3% (12). Pinprick hyperalgesia was present in 57%, cold allodynia in 40%, and brush-evoked dysesthesia in 51% of affected patients.

The thalamic syndrome was first described by Dejerine and Roussy (13). The onset of pain is usually delayed (1–3 months after the stoke), but can also be a sign of acute stroke (14) as in this patient where pain was among the acute symptoms. The hand is most frequently afflicted in thalamic pain. All pain qualities may be involved (1). There are no pathognomonic features. Descriptors used for spontaneous pain are burning, aching, pricking, freezing, and squeezing; intermittent pain is often described as lancinating or shooting (4). Central pain resulting from posterior parasylvian lesions has been suggested as a separate entity characterized by burning or aching pain with allodynia (15).

The pathophysiology of central pain is controversial. Partial injury to the spinothalamic pathway seems to involve a greater risk for central pain than complete injury (16). Mechanisms discussed have included abnormal hypersensitivity of central neurons and fibers, alterations in impulse patterns, and activation of silent synapses. The thermosensory disinhibition theory states that central post-stroke pain is due to loss of normal inhibition of cold pain. In this hypothesis, there is an imbalance between a lateral spinothalamic tract involved in signaling the feeling of cold and a medial spinothalamic tract signaling pain (4). A disturbance of GABAergic neurotransmission between the sensory thalamus and sensory cortical areas has also been suggested (17).

References

(1) Bowsher D, Leijon G, Thuomas KA. Central poststroke pain: correlation of MRI with clinical pain characteristics and sensory abnormalities. *Neurology* 1998;51:1352–1358.

(2) Schmahmann JD. Vascular syndromes of the thalamus. *Stroke* 2003;34:2264–2278.

(3) Boivie J. Central pain. In: McMahon SB, Koltzenburg M, eds. *Textbook of Pain*. Edinburgh: Churchill Livingstone, 2006:1057–1074.

(4) Klit H, Finnerup NB, Jensen TS. Central post-stroke pain: clinical characteristics, pathophysiology, and management. *Lancet Neurol* 2009;8:857–868.

(5) Leijon G, Boivie J. Central post-stroke pain–a controlled trial of amitriptyline and carbamazepine. *Pain* 1989;36:27–36.

(6) Vestergaard K, Andersen G, Gottrup H, Kristensen BT, Jensen TS. Lamotrigine for central poststroke pain: a randomized controlled trial. *Neurology* 2001;56:184–190.

(7) Kim JS, Bashford G, Murphy TK, Martin A, Dror V, Cheung R. Safety and efficacy of pregabalin in patients with central post-stroke pain. *Pain* 2011; 152:1018–1023.

(8) Eisenberg E, McNicol ED, Carr DB. Efficacy and safety of opioid agonists in the treatment of neuropathic pain of nonmalignant origin: systematic review and meta-analysis of randomized controlled trials. *JAMA* 2005;293:3043–3052.

(9) Tasker RR. History of lesioning for pain. *Stereotact Funct Neurosurg* 2001;77:163–165.

(10) Nandi D, Smith H, Owen S, Joint C, Stein J, Aziz T. Peri-ventricular grey stimulation versus motor cortex stimulation for post stroke neuropathic pain. *J Clin Neurosci* 2002;9:557–561.

(11) Yamamoto T, Katayama Y, Hirayama T, Tsubokawa T. Pharmacological classification of central post-stroke pain: comparison with the results of chronic motor cortex stimulation therapy. *Pain* 1997;72:5–12.

(12) Klit H, Finnerup NB, Andersen G, Jensen TS. Central poststroke pain: a population-based study. *Pain* 2011;152:818–824.

(13) Dejerine J, Roussy G. Le syndrome thalamique. *Rev Neurol* 1906;14:521–532.

(14) Paciaroni M, Bogousslavsky J. Pure sensory syndromes in thalamic stroke. *Eur Neurol* 1998;39:211–217.

(15) Garcia-Larrea L, Perchet C, Creac'h C, et al. Operculo-insular pain (parasylvian pain): a distinct central pain syndrome. *Brain* 2010;133:2528–2539.

(16) Hong JH, Choi BY, Chang CH, et al. The prevalence of central poststroke pain according to the integrity of the spino-thalamo-cortical pathway. *Eur Neurol* 2012;67:12–17.

(17) Canavero S, Bonicalzi V. Central pain syndrome: elucidation of genesis and treatment. *Expert Rev Neurother* 2007;7:1485–1497.

Pain in multiple sclerosis

Whether pain is more frequent in patients with multiple sclerosis (MS) than in the general population has been debated. Independent of this question, it is worth knowing the special characteristics of pain in MS and the available treatment options.

Clinical case vignette

A 30-year-old female experienced her first symptoms of MS when she noticed numbness of her palms. No neurological diagnosis was made, but the patient was found to suffer from bipolar affective disorder. Her history included one suicide attempt with the use of antidepressant drugs. Her family history was positive for depression. Five years later, a diagnosis of relapsing-remitting MS was confirmed when the patient presented with hemiparesis on the right that improved while she received a course of corticosteroid treatment. Treatment with Interferon-ß1b was initiated. She developed slowly progressive weakness and spasticity of both legs 2 years later and a secondary progressive disease course was diagnosed. In the same year, the patient also reported an intermittent electric-shock–like pain in the left jaw. There were weeks when she experienced this pain with almost every movement of the facial muscles, and other periods when she was almost pain free. A diagnosis of trigeminal neuralgia was made, and carbamazepine, administered up to a dose of 800 mg/day, provided some pain relief. Additional MS symptoms developed in the next 2 years, including bladder disturbance and ataxia. The patient underwent repeated pulse therapies with high-dose methylprednisolone, but these did not noticeably improve her motor symptoms and had no effect on the pain. Over time, the patient developed other types of intermittent pain that could last for months, followed by some degree of remission. One prominent complaint was Lhermitte's sign which the patient did not classify as painful but as very disturbing. She sometimes presented with back pain, headache, or a continuous burning pain in both legs which was worse at night. While she could cope with most of these symptoms, she regularly saw a neurologist for the pain associated with her trigeminal neuralgia. When carbamazepine appeared to lose its effect, treatment was changed to lamotrigine, which was slowly increased to 100 mg bid. With her MS being confirmed as being secondary chronic progressive, the patient's basic therapy was changed to mitoxantrone at 3-monthly applications. This was stopped after three applications because of toxic cardiomyopathy. The trigeminal pain worsened again, and the patient was hardly able to speak, eat, or drink without provoking pain attacks. Lamotrigine was stopped and carbamazepine was initiated again, this time up to 1200 mg/day. This dose provided some pain relief, but the patient suffered from severe fatigue and believed that her ataxia had become even worse. She was referred to the Department of Neurosurgery for evaluation. Cranial MRI showed multiple MS lesions [Figure 26.1] although none were specific to the area of the trigeminal nucleus. Vascular compression of the trigeminal nerve entry zone into the pons was not detected. Despite this finding and supported by case reports in the literature (1), a trigeminovascular decompression (Jannetta operation) was performed. There were no perioperative complications. Immediately post-operatively the patient reported that the pain attacks had stopped. While convalescing on the neurosurgical ward, no further attacks occurred. Carbamazepine was slowly tapered to 150 mg bid over the next 2 months. While there were no further episodes of pain, the patient, fearful of recurrence, did not wish to have the dose reduced any further.

Nine months later, she came to the Emergency Department with complaints of increasing facial pain attacks on the left. The pain attacks had changed in character. Still in the same location, they currently lasted up to 30 min in duration and produced a burning sensation. She reported that attempts to increase

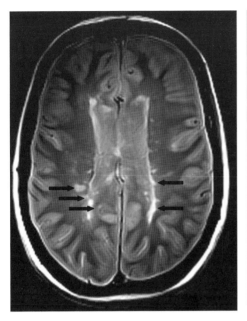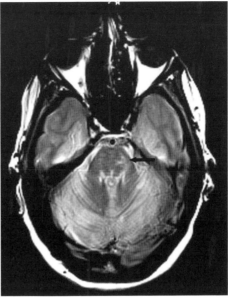

Figure 26.1. (left) MRI scan at the height of the lateral ventricles showing multiple periventrical lesions (arrows), typical in MS. (right) Pontine lesion (arrow), potentially responsible for trigeminal neuralgia in this patient. Courtesy of Prof. Solymosi, Department of Neuroradiology, University Hospital of Würzburg.

the carbamazepine dose had aggravated her condition. Low-dose pregabalin was added to her drug therapy but this also increased her pain. She was very anxious and often agitated. When asked about her pain level, she could not precisely describe it and believed that she was more handicapped by the fear of pain than by the pain itself. She requested further neurosurgical input but further intervention was declined. The patient subsequently admitted herself to a psychiatric hospital where she was stabilized and experienced reasonable health in the following months. When she reported again to our outpatient department, she clearly stated that the facial pain attacks were related to stress or anxiety and that her use of relaxation techniques was helpful. She had stopped all medication related to trigeminal neuralgia. She was able to walk with an ambulator in her home and used a wheelchair out-of-doors. She still had intermittent painful spasms in her legs, Lhermitte's sign on bending the head, and dysesthesias of the legs. These symptoms annoyed her but she did not want any specific treatment for them.

Pain description

The patient's original pain attacks of stabbing and electric-shock–like character in the distribution of one or two branches of the trigeminal nerve are characteristic of trigeminal neuralgia. The attacks could be brief, lasting only for a few seconds, or they could persist for up to 30 min in duration. Pain attacks were induced by touching the skin, talking, eating, and brushing the teeth. After the pain-free period following the Jannetta operation, the quality of the pain changed. Attacks were no longer brief but generally lasted up to 30 min and produced a burning sensation. They were less dependent upon touch or facial movement and appeared related to the patient's emotional or psychological state.

The other, less severe pains and dysesthesias the patient suffered from were Lhermitte's sign, a tingling feeling running down her spine when she bent her head, and painful leg spasms that were dependent on the degree of spasticity at a certain time point. Furthermore, she had a variable leg pain that sometimes manifested as a continuous burning pain, sometimes as dysesthesia with a tingling and mildly burning sensation.

Pain in multiple sclerosis

The epidemiology and the characteristics of pain in patients with MS have been described in several large

109

cohorts. The resulting estimates of pain prevalence have ranged between 29 and 86% of MS patients. A systematic review identified a point prevalence of pain of nearly 50% (2). The presence of pain was associated with increased age, duration of illness, depression, degree of functional impairment, and fatigue. Pain reporting by MS patients may be similar to that reported by the general population but MS patients are more likely to have severe pain, to use analgesics, or to suffer from interference with activities of daily living (3). Pain is associated with poorer quality of life in MS patients and most prominently affects physical and emotional functioning (2). Older patients, those with longer disease duration and greater disease severity have a higher likelihood to suffer from pain. There seems to be no gender difference in the prevalence of pain, but women report a greater severity. There is a higher risk of developing pain in chronic progressive types than in relapsing-remitting MS (4). Clinical data suggest that only patients with lesions in the spinothalamo-cortical pathways run the risk of developing central pain (5, 6). In contrast, localization of the inflammatory/demyelinating lesions specifically within the pain pathway on MRI scans was not associated with increased pain (7).

In a cross-sectional study involving 1672 Italian patients (4), the most frequent pain complaint was dysesthetic pain with 18%, followed by back pain, painful spams, and Lhermitte's sign. Trigeminal neuralgia occurred only in 2% of patients. In Portuguese MS patients, the prevalence of pain was 34%, with headache and back pain being the most common sites (8). It has been hypothesized that, like in other chronic pain, a biopsychosocial perspective should be taken in MS (9). In the patient cohort studied by these authors, pain was present in 82%. Interestingly, pain intensity correlated only with physical aspects, whereas quality of pain was additionally associated with increased avoidance, resignation, and fatigue.

Patients with MS may suffer from several different types of pain, including central pain, extremity pain, trigeminal neuralgia, Lhermitte's sign, painful tonic spasms, back pain, and headache (2). The following classification of pain in MS has been suggested: 1. continuous central neuropathic pain, 2. intermittent central neuropathic pain, 3. musculoskeletal pain, 4. mixed neuropathic and non-neuropathic pain (2). Central pain is assumed if the distribution of pain is consistent with a central nervous system lesion, and if a thorough evaluation for alternative nociceptive

and peripheral neuropathic pain and psychiatric disease is negative (6). The most common pain qualities in a series of 100 patients with MS and central pain were burning and aching. The most common central neuropathic pain conditions in patients with MS are extremity pain, trigeminal neuralgia, and Lhermitte's sign. Extremity pain is usually chronic and described as a continuous burning pain which is often bilateral, worse at night, and exacerbated during physical activity. It is thought to derive from lesions in the spinal cord leading to dysfunction of inhibitory GABAergic interneurons.

Trigeminal neuralgia, with a prevalence of 1–2%, is 20 times more common in MS patients than in the general population. This condition has also been labeled "atypical facial pain" associated with MS. MS patients, on average, are much younger than patients with classical trigeminal neuralgia. Also, approximately 20% of cases with trigeminal neuralgia are bilateral in MS patients, which is much more than in the general population. It may be the presenting symptom of MS (10). Lesions at the trigeminal nerve entry zone are present in some patients, although similar lesions have been reported in patients without trigeminal pain (11, 12). Even lesions in the trigeminal root itself have been described, but only in a few case series (13, 14). This has also been confirmed in autopsy cases.

Lhermitte's sign is caused by demyelinating lesions in the posterior columns of the cervical spinal cord (15), which lead to hypersensitivity of cervical sensory axons to stretching. In prospective studies, Lhermitte's sign has been present at some point during the disease course in 40% of patients (2). Patients usually report that they can elicit the symptom by neck flexion and describe its character as electric-shock – like or tingling. The duration is short, lasting only a few seconds. Lhermitte' sign, once it appears, may remit within 4–6 weeks but it may also recur or become chronic.

Many MS patients suffer from spasticity, but this is not necessarily painful. Some patients have painful tonic spasms lasting a few minutes, which may occur several times per day. They can be triggered by touch, movement, or strong emotions. In the past, these spasms have also been called "brainstem seizures," but there are no data confirming the epileptic character of these spasms.

The frequency of headache, in particular migraine, seems to be increased in MS patients. This has been associated with lesions in the midbrain (16). Secondary musculoskeletal pain may also develop in MS patients, possibly due to weakness, muscle spasms, spasticity, and reduced mobility. Secondary musculoskeletal pain can manifest in the form of back pain or extremity pain. Chronic steroid use can cause osteoporosis with a risk of compression fractures.

It is unclear whether disease-modifying treatment improves the pain. Pain is not a primary outcome in most clinical trials involving MS. There are transient increases of pain in the first month of treatment with interferon beta (17). Interferon beta and glatiramer acetate treatment may be associated with an increased incidence of headaches, especially in patients with a history of headaches (18).

Few trials have explicitly tested the effects of drugs to treat pain in MS (19). Of those, five have tested the effect of cannabinoids. The results of these trials suggest that cannabinoids may be effective in some patients with MS pain, but confirmatory trials are needed. Furthermore, there are concerns about the long-term safety of these drugs, including the risk of precipitating psychosis or schizophrenia, especially in individuals with environmental or genetic risk factors (2).

Gabapentin has been suggested as first-line treatment for patients with spasticity-related pain because of its good safety profile (20). Oral baclofen and cannabinoids are regarded as second-line drugs. Intrathecal baclofen can be used for patients with severe spasticity resistant to oral drugs. In painful tonic spasms, gabapentin and pregabalin produced pain relief in open-label studies. Lamotrigine was effective in improving pain in five of eight patients with painful tonic spasms. Orally administered sodium channel blockers such as carbamazepine are also recommended. Trigeminal neuropathy can be treated with carbamazepine, oxcarbazepine, or lamotrigine. The response rate to sodium channel blockers seems to be lower than in classical trigeminal neuralgia. Gabapentin and topiramate may be alternatives. Misoprostol, a prostaglandin-E1-analog that targets the MS-related inflammatory mechanisms, was effective in two small studies. Experts recommend treatment of MS-related trigeminal neuralgia along the guidelines for classical trigeminal neuralgia (19–21). Lhermitte's sign is not often specifically treated. Should treatment be required, orally administered sodium-channel blockers such as carbamazepine or oxcarbazepine may be offered. Central neuropathic pain can be treated with tricyclic antidepressants, gabapentin,

or lamotrigine; there are insufficient data however to definitely prove efficacy or the preference of one drug over another (19, 20). In summary, pain treatment in MS remains an individual decision. The potential side-effects of therapeutic regimes and their impact on quality of life must be carefully weighed.

References

(1) Broggi G, Ferroli P, Franzini A, et al. Operative findings and outcomes of microvascular decompression for trigeminal neuralgia in 35 patients affected by multiple sclerosis. *Neurosurgery* 2004;55:830–838; discussion 838–839.

(2) O'Connor AB, Schwid SR, Herrmann DN, Markman JD, Dworkin RH. Pain associated with multiple sclerosis: systematic review and proposed classification. *Pain* 2008;137:96–111.

(3) Svendsen KB, Jensen TS, Overvad K, Hansen HJ, Koch-Henriksen N, Bach FW. Pain in patients with multiple sclerosis: a population-based study. *Arch Neurol* 2003;60:1089–1094.

(4) Solaro C, Brichetto G, Amato MP, et al. The prevalence of pain in multiple sclerosis: a multicenter cross-sectional study. *Neurology* 2004;63:919–921.

(5) Osterberg A, Boivie J. Central pain in multiple sclerosis – sensory abnormalities. *Eur J Pain* 2010;14:104–110.

(6) Osterberg A, Boivie J, Thuomas KA. Central pain in multiple sclerosis – prevalence and clinical characteristics. *Eur J Pain* 2005;9:531–542.

(7) Svendsen KB, Sorensen L, Jensen TS, Hansen HJ, Bach FW. MRI of the central nervous system in MS patients with and without pain. *Eur J Pain* 2011; 15:395–401.

(8) Seixas D, Sa MJ, Galhardo V, Guimaraes J, Lima D. Pain in Portuguese patients with multiple sclerosis. *Front Neurol* 2011;2:20.

(9) Michalski D, Liebig S, Thomae E, Hinz A, Bergh FT. Pain in patients with multiple sclerosis: a complex assessment including quantitative and qualitative measurements provides for a disease-related biopsychosocial pain model. *J Pain Res* 2011;4: 219–225.

(10) Hooge JP, Redekop WK. Trigeminal neuralgia in multiple sclerosis. *Neurology* 1995;45:1294–1296.

(11) da Silva CJ, da Rocha AJ, Mendes MF, et al. Trigeminal involvement in multiple sclerosis: magnetic resonance imaging findings with clinical correlation in a series of patients. *Mult Scler* 2005;11:282–285.

(12) Gass A, Kitchen N, MacManus DG, Moseley IF, Hennerici MG, Miller DH. Trigeminal neuralgia in patients with multiple sclerosis: lesion localization with magnetic resonance imaging. *Neurology* 1997;49:1142–1144.

(13) Ferroli P, Farina L, Franzini A, Milanese C, Broggi G. Linear pontine and trigeminal root lesions and trigeminal neuralgia. *Arch Neurol* 2001;58:1311–1312.

(14) Nakashima I, Fujihara K, Kimpara T, Okita N, Takase S, Itoyama Y. Linear pontine trigeminal root lesions in multiple sclerosis: clinical and magnetic resonance imaging studies in 5 cases. *Arch Neurol* 2001;58: 101–104.

(15) Gutrecht JA, Zamani AA, Slagado ED. Anatomic-radiologic basis of Lhermitte's sign in multiple sclerosis. *Arch Neurol* 1993;50:849–851.

(16) Gee JR, Chang J, Dublin AB, Vijayan N. The association of brainstem lesions with migraine-like headache: an imaging study of multiple sclerosis. *Headache* 2005;45:670–677.

(17) Arnoldus JH, Killestein J, Pfennings LE, Jelles B, Uitdehaag BM, Polman CH. Quality of life during the first 6 months of interferon-beta treatment in patients with MS. *Mult Scler* 2000;6:338–342.

(18) Pöllmann W, Erasmus LP, Feneberg W, Straube A. The effect of glatiramer acetate treatment on pre-existing headaches in patients with MS. *Neurology* 2006;66:275–277.

(19) Solaro C, Uccelli MM. Management of pain in multiple sclerosis: a pharmacological approach. *Nat Rev Neurol* 2011;7:519–527.

(20) Truini A, Galeotti F, Cruccu G. Treating pain in multiple sclerosis. *Expert Opin Pharmacother* 2011;12:2355–2368.

(21) Cruccu G, Gronseth G, Alksne J, et al. AAN-EFNS guidelines on trigeminal neuralgia management. *Eur J Neurol* 2008;15:1013–1028.

Chapter 27

Chronic migraine

The prevalence of migraine is approximately 6% in men and 15% in women. While episodic migraine is adequately treated with analgesics or triptans that stop a migraine attack, the therapeutic management of chronic migraine can be challenging.

Clinical case vignette

A 49-year-old female reported that she had suffered migraine attacks since age 25. Her family history included a brother and son with the same affliction. For many years, the migraine occurred approximately once per week. The patient was able to abort the attacks with aspirin or a combination of aspirin and paracetamol. Attacks were described as one sided but the side varied. The headache was pulsating, became more severe upon movement, and reached a severity of 8/10. Most attacks were accompanied by nausea. If the attacks were severe, and in particular if the patient were unable to take her analgesic within a specific time-frame, vomiting occurred. These attacks were also accompanied by severe sensitivity to light, noise, and also smells. During severe attacks, the patient felt compelled to lie down. If she managed to fall asleep, the attacks were usually gone the next morning. Five years previously with attacks occurring at a rate of 4 per month, the patient had been prescribed a beta-blocker for prophylaxis. She experienced no improvement and terminated the drug after 8 weeks. Acupuncture with an accredited physician was attempted with no beneficial results. After 3 months, this was also terminated. The patient resolved to live with her once weekly migraine attack by taking an analgesic in the early stages of an attack and hopefully, becoming pain free within a few hours.

In the past 2 years, the patient began to experience more frequent, even daily migraine attacks. Simple analgesics were no longer effective, and the patient began using a triptan (sumatriptan). Upon examination at the migraine clinic, she reported taking approx-imately 20 tablets of sumatriptan per month, and having very few headache-free days. She was still able to abort the attacks by medicating herself quickly and as a result had good work attendance with few sick days. Increasingly, she had noticed a background headache between migraine attacks. She had always been athletic and until the onset of this second headache, had managed to run three times a week, finding that regular exercise reduced the frequency of her migraines. Due to the ongoing nature of the headache, she was forced to reduce her physical activity and had gained 20 kg over 2 years.

At the time of consultation, the patient suffered from a headache of intermediate severity. On examination, her head was sensitive to percussion and the pericranial musculature was hyperalgesic to pressure. Her neurological examination was otherwise normal.

The patient was advised to use a headache diary (Table 27.1) and given options for migraine prophylaxis. She opted against ß-blockers because of their past ineffectiveness. After informed consent, she agreed to try topiramate, a second drug designed and licensed for migraine prophylaxis. She was made aware of frequently encountered side-effects including tingling of the hands, changes in taste of carbonated drinks, irritability, depression, and weight loss. The initial dose of topiramate was 25 mg with a weekly increase of 25 mg to a maintenance dose of 50 mg bid. The patient was reassessed 3 months later. She had noticed a marked decline in headache days and triptan intake since being on the maintenance dose of topiramate. For the first time in years, she had headache-free stretches lasting up to 10 days [Table 27.1].

Pain description

The IHC criteria for migraine are pulsating headaches accompanied by two of the following: nausea, vomiting, and sensitivity to noise and light. Our patient fulfilled these criteria. Her additional complaint of a more

Table 27.1. Headache diary recorded from the patient described in this vignette

	Jan	Feb	March	April	May	June	July
1	MTT	H		H			MTT
2	MT	H	MTT	H			MT
3	H	MTT	MTT	H	H		H
4	H	MTT	MTT		H		H
5		H	MT	M	H		
6	MTT	H	MT	M			
7	MTT		H	H		H	
8	M			H	M	H	
9		MTT	MTT		M	H	
10	MTT	MTT	MTT		H	M	
11	MTT	MTT	H	MT		H	
12	H	MTT	H	MT	MTT	H	
13	H	MT	H	H	MT		
14	MTT	MT		H	MT	M	M
15	MTT	H	MT		H	M	H
16	MTT	H	MT			H	H
17			H				
18	MTT	MTT	H	H	H		
19	H	MTT	H	H	H		
20	M	H		M	M	MT	
21	MT	M		MTT		H	
22	MT	MT	M	M		H	MT
23	H	M	MTT	H	H		M
24	H	H	MTT		H		H
25	H	H	MTT		H	H	
26	MT	MTT	H	H	H	H	
27	MT	MTT	H	H	H	H	H
28	M		H	H		H	H
29				H		H	H
30	H		H	H		H	
31	H		H				
No sumatriptan tablets	23	21	20	4	4	1	4
Start topiramate							

M: migraine attack; T: one sumatriptan tablet; H: headache.

continuous headache interspersed with headaches that increased in severity and which the patient believed to be migraines was of interest. She described the former as being of intermediate severity, pressure-like, and involving the entire skull. In addition, the difference in severity between the two types had become smaller.

Discussion

The condition of chronic migraine was initially termed "transformed migraine" (1). It denoted patients with medication overuse as well as patients whose ailment had completely changed (transformed) to resemble a tension headache. The second edition of the International Classification of Headache Disorders (2) adopted the term chronic migraine. Chronic migraine was initially defined as migraine without aura for 15 or more days per month for longer than 3 months and in the absence of medication overuse. For several reasons, this definition was unhelpful in clinical practice. Many patients with chronic migraine can use considerable amounts of medication. The headache character changes when migraine becomes chronic, and finally, migraine headaches do not share the same characteristics. Thus, the definition of chronic migraine has changed over time. The revised definition requires 15 or more headache days per month, of which 8 or more fulfill the migraine criteria (3). Of note, a change in headache character is an indication for brain imaging so that causes of secondary headache can be excluded (4). The current definition of chronic migraine includes cases with medication overuse, but this should be separately noted because it changes the treatment approach (5). Patients are required to experience typical migraine headache during at least 8 of their 15 or more headache days per month. Migraine can be diagnosed if the headache is unilateral, of moderate to severe intensity, pulsating, and aggravated by physical activity. At least two of these characteristics must be present. Combined associated symptoms (nausea and/or vomiting, photophobia, and phonophobia) are required.

The reported prevalence of chronic migraine is 1.4–2.2% in the overall population (6). Patients with episodic migraine have an annual risk of 2.5% of developing chronic migraine (7). An intermediate headache frequency of 6 to 9 days per month and in particular, a critical frequency of 10 to 14 headache days per month, increase the risk for chronicity (8). Additional risk factors include obesity, stressful life events, snoring, and overuse of certain classes of medication. The use of barbiturates and opiates is associated with an increased risk of developing chronic migraine (9).

The differential diagnosis of chronic migraine includes other primary headache disorders with attacks of long duration. Chronic tension-type headache can be differentiated from chronic migraine by its character. It is usually bilateral, not pulsating, and of mild to moderate intensity. It is not aggravated by physical activity. The associated symptoms of migraine like photophobia, phonophobia, nausea, and vomiting are not present, or, if so, only mildly and not in combination (2). Another differential diagnosis is new daily persistent headache. Here, the headache is unremitting from onset or within 3 days of onset (2). The presence of more than one migrainous feature (photophobia, phonophobia, nausea) precludes this diagnosis. The other primary chronic headache, hemicrania continua, manifests with unilateral pain like most migraine attacks. The pain is continuous, but there may be phases of moderate intensity and exacerbations of high intensity, which may resemble an attack. Because nausea and photophobia may occur in hemicrania continua, it may be mistaken for migraine. It does not respond to either acute or prophylactic migraine drugs but notably, indomethacin is effective. Thus, the hallmark of hemicrania continua, the presence of ipsilateral autonomic symptoms including lacrimation, conjunctival injection, ptosis, and rhinorrhea, must be carefully assessed.

Chronic migraine is a dynamic entity. In a recent study on the evolution of chronic migraine, 26% of patients re-experienced episodic migraine and 34% had persistent chronic migraine (10). Age of onset or depression status were not related factors. More patients without prophylactic medication began experiencing episodic migraine again. Also, more patients with severe allodynia had persistent chronic migraine. A further negative predictor of remission was a high frequency rate, i.e., attacks occurring 25–31 days per month. Finally, another study demonstrates that compliance to preventive medication is a factor in favor of reversion to episodic migraine (11).

Like other chronic pain disorders, chronic migraine is associated with several comorbidities such as depression, anxiety, disorders of the heart and of the respiratory system (5). Most of these are also associated with episodic migraine, but the incidence is much higher in chronic migraine. This relationship is also supported by the migraine disability assessment scale (MIDAS) which assesses the level of patient disability. Here, patients with episodic migraine reach a score of 10, those with chronic migraine in contrast have a score of 63 (5).

Pain in chronic migraine

Structural, functional, and pharmacologic changes have been implicated in the pathophysiology of chronic migraine (12). As in other chronic pain disorders, decreased areas of gray matter in several brain regions involved in pain processing have been found. Iron deposition in the basal ganglia and thus an increased accumulation of iron in the antinociceptive network appear to have a role in migraine chronification or possibly physiological response to repeated activation of brain areas involved in central pain processing (13). Increased cortical excitability was demonstrated in patients with chronic migraine using transcranial magnetic stimulation combined with positron emission tomography (PET) (12). The allodynia often observed in patients with chronic migraine is interpreted as an indication of central sensitization, i.e., CNS involvement is stronger in chronic as opposed to episodic migraine.

As in episodic migraine, individual attacks can be treated with triptans. However, triptans should not be taken for more than 9 days per month. The risk for chronic misuse of triptans becomes significant with its use of 12 days or more per month (7). Non-pharmacologic measures to reduce headache frequency include regular exercise, relaxation techniques such as progressive muscular relaxation, and acupuncture. Regular exercise (exercise for more than 3 times a week for more than 30 min at a time) is one of the factors favoring remission of chronic migraine (11).

The drugs available for prophylactic treatment of migraine are derived from very different substance groups but have one point in common. All of them experimentally reduce cortical spreading depression, a factor thought to be central to migraine pathogenesis. This was shown for propranolol, topiramate, valproate, amitriptyline, and methysergide (14). Of these, topiramate in particular was used in a trial with chronic migraine (15). Subcutaneous botulinum toxin, which also reduced headache days in patients with chronic migraine (16), is assumed to reduce peripheral sensitization. Prophylactic medication is recommended in all patients with chronic migraine to reduce suffering and to avoid potential long-term sequelae (17).

The impact of prophylactic medication observed in the patient described above is among the most favorable ones in the author's experience. It is unlikely that the rapid decline in triptan use was caused by the prophylactic medication alone. The successful resolution to this case may also be attributed to educating the patient about the problems of chronic migraine and medication overuse. The combination of patient information, attention to her needs, and care plus the preventive medication may all have been of benefit.

References

(1) Mathew NT, Stubits E, Nigam MP. Transformation of episodic migraine into daily headache: analysis of factors. *Headache* 1982;22:66–68.

(2) Headache Classification Subcommittee of the International Headache Society. The International Classification of Headache Disorders. 2nd edition. *Cephalalgia* 2004;24(Suppl 1):9–160.

(3) Katsarava Z, Manack A, Yoon MS, et al. Chronic migraine: classification and comparisons. *Cephalalgia* 2011;31:520–529.

(4) Silberstein SD. Practice parameter: evidence-based guidelines for migraine headache (an evidence-based review): report of the Quality Standards Subcommittee of the American Academy of Neurology. *Neurology* 2000;55:754–762.

(5) Lipton RB. Chronic migraine, classification, differential diagnosis, and epidemiology. *Headache* 2011;51(Suppl 2):77–83.

(6) Natoli JL, Manack A, Dean B, et al. Global prevalence of chronic migraine: a systematic review. *Cephalalgia* 2010;30:599–609.

(7) Bigal ME, Serrano D, Buse D, Scher A, Stewart WF, Lipton RB. Acute migraine medications and evolution from episodic to chronic migraine: a longitudinal population-based study. *Headache* 2008;48:1157–1168.

(8) Lipton RB. Tracing transformation: chronic migraine classification, progression, and epidemiology. *Neurology* 2009;72:S3–S7.

(9) Bigal ME, Lipton RB. Concepts and mechanisms of migraine chronification. *Headache* 2008;48:7–15.

(10) Manack A, Buse DC, Serrano D, Turkel CC, Lipton RB. Rates, predictors, and consequences of remission from chronic migraine to episodic migraine. *Neurology* 2011;76:711–718.

(11) Seok JI, Cho HI, Chung CS. From transformed migraine to episodic migraine: reversion factors. *Headache* 2006;46:1186–1190.

(12) Mathew NT. Pathophysiology of chronic migraine and mode of action of preventive medications. *Headache* 2011;51(Suppl 2):84–92.

(13) Kruit MC, Launer LJ, Overbosch J, van Buchem MA, Ferrari MD. Iron accumulation in deep brain nuclei in migraine: a population-based magnetic resonance imaging study. *Cephalalgia* 2009;29:351–359.

(14) Ayata C, Jin H, Kudo C, Dalkara T, Moskowitz MA. Suppression of cortical spreading depression in migraine prophylaxis. *Ann Neurol* 2006;59:652–661.

(15) Diener HC, Bussone G, Van Oene JC, Lahaye M, Schwalen S, Goadsby PJ. Topiramate reduces

headache days in chronic migraine: a randomized, double-blind, placebo-controlled study. *Cephalalgia* 2007;27:814–823.

(16) Diener HC, Dodick DW, Aurora SK, et al. OnabotulinumtoxinA for treatment of chronic migraine: results from the double-blind, randomized, placebo-controlled phase of the PREEMPT 2 trial. *Cephalalgia* 2010;30:804–814.

(17) Evers S, Afra J, Frese A, et al. EFNS guideline on the drug treatment of migraine – revised report of an EFNS task force. *Eur J Neurol* 2009;16: 968–981.

Chapter

28

Cluster headache

Cluster headache is one of several primary headache conditions. In contrast to most other headaches, it primarily targets men. Patients suffer from attacks of excruciating pain, which present in a specific temporal pattern.

Clinical case vignette

A 41-year-old man was seen at the headache clinic in October 2011 complaining of pain attacks which had woken him with uncanny punctuality at 2 a.m for the past 15 nights. His descriptions localized the attacks to the right orbit and were of such extreme severity that he felt compelled to leave his bed and pace in his room. Asked about the quality of his pain, the patient stated it was as if someone had pushed his eyeball out from behind or someone had stabbed a hot dagger through his eye [Figure 28.1]. He spoke of suicidal ideation during these attacks. Upon questioning, he also reported reddening and tearing in his right eye as well as "runniness" in the right nostril. The attacks always occurred on the same side and usually lasted between 30 and 60 min. Afterward, he still experienced a dull pain on the right side of his head, but was able to resume sleeping. Other than feeling fatigued, he had no other symptoms on the following mornings. His use of over-the-counter analgesics included ibuprofen and paracetamol but neither relieved the pain. Because the durations of the attacks were limited to approximately 1 h, he wondered if the analgesics might have had some effect.

When asked for previous headache experiences, the patient reported that he had suffered from a similar episode approximately 2 years previously. At that time, the attacks had also been very severe, although not as excruciating as his current attacks. The episode had lasted approximately 10 or 12 days, and he had not consulted a physician. The patient's history was otherwise unremarkable. He had never been seriously ill. He occasionally suffered from mild headaches, likely due

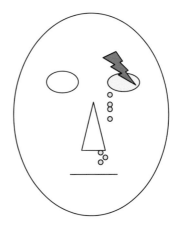

Figure 28.1. Drawing including the main symptoms of a cluster headache attack: Very severe pain in the region of the orbit, conjunctival injection, lacrimation, and rhinorrhea.

to stress at work or alcohol consumption, which readily responded to ibuprofen. They occurred during the day, were holocephalic and of dull quality, and had no other associated symptoms. They did not impact his activities, whether work related or otherwise. They usually lasted for several hours and were alleviated by either ibuprofen or by vigorous walking in fresh air. There was no family history of migraine or other headache disorders. As an accountant, he had a sedentary occupation but exercised in his free time and felt reasonably fit. He was a cigarette smoker and drank moderate amounts of wine and beer.

The patient was informed that his headache fulfilled the criteria for cluster headache and the treatment options were discussed. He remained in the hospital overnight for a trial of oxygen treatment which resulted in abortion of his attack within 10 min. He was discharged with a prescription of subcutaneous sumatriptan for self-application should further attacks occur. The patient's attacks did return, and the sumatriptan alleviated his symptoms within 15 min. In addition, a dose of 1 mg/kg of oral prednisolone was initiated and the patient was instructed to reduce the dose once the nightly attacks ended. After a few nights with milder attacks, the attacks ceased and the prednisolone was tapered over 3 weeks. At a follow-up visit 3 months later, the patient was free of headache complaints.

Pain description

The patient described his pain as very severe, excruciating, and worse than anything he had experienced before. Asked to rate the pain on a scale of 0 to 10, he chose "12." He could not attribute any of the standard pain qualities (burning, pulsating, dull, etc.) to his experience, but instead used very vivid descriptions and analogies. For example, the pain felt as if someone was pushing the eyeball out from behind or splitting his skull at the site of his orbit with a burning dagger. He admitted to suicidal ideations during the attacks. Standard analgesics had no effect. The pain attacks woke him up from sleep, and he felt compelled to get up and walk about, although this by no means reduced the pain intensity. The patient also reported associated symptoms such as reddening and lacrimation of the ipsilateral eye and rhinorrhea.

Discussion

Cluster headache is a distinct clinical syndrome already described in detail by Nicolas Tulp in the 17th century (1). Following the observations of Bayard T. Horton, a neurologist in North America, the syndrome became known as Horton headache (1). It is currently classified among the trigeminal autonomic cephalalgias. The term cluster headache is derived from the periodicity of the attacks which occur in "clusters" and then remit for various time spans.

The International Headache Society (IHS) has defined this syndrome as severe or very severe unilateral orbital, supraorbital and/or temporal pain lasting 15–180 min if untreated, accompanied either by ipsilateral conjunctival injection or lacrimation, ipsilateral nasal congestion or rhinorrhea, ipsilateral eyelid edema, ipsilateral miosis, or ptosis or a sense of restlessness or agitation [Table 28.1]. Most patients experience combinations of these symptoms. Additional mandatory criteria are a frequency of attacks of one in 2 days to eight per day and the exclusion of other causative disorders.

Cluster headache has an estimated prevalence of 0.1% in the general population (2). Men are affected more than women in a ratio of approximately 4 to 1. The mean age of initial presentation is 30 years. Onset in childhood is possible (3). There is a familial com-

Table 28.1. Criteria for cluster headache according to the International Headache Society (IHS) (22)

At least 5 attacks fulfilling the following criteria:
Severe or very severe unilateral orbital, supraorbital, or temporal pain lasting 15 to 180 min if untreated.
Headache accompanied by one of the following:
– ipsilateral conjunctival infection or lacrimation
– ipsilateral nasal congestion or rhinorrhea
– ipsilateral eyelid edema
– ipsilateral forehead and facial sweating
– ipsilateral miosis or ptosis
– a sense of restlessness or agitation
Attacks have a frequency from one every other day to 8 per day
Attacks are not attributed to another disorder

Episodic cluster headache: at least two cluster periods lasting 7 days to 1 year and separated by pain-free remission periods of 1 month or more; chronic cluster headache: attacks that recur for more than 1 year, without remission periods or with remission periods lasting less than 1 month.

ponent, but specific genes have not been identified. Lifestyle plays an important role (4). Patients with cluster headache are typically smokers and have frequent alcohol intake.

Cluster headache must be differentiated from the other trigemino-autonomic syndromes. All exhibit short-lasting, unilateral, severe headache attacks with ipsilateral autonomic symptoms. The main differences are those of duration and frequency of attacks. In paroxysmal hemicrania, women are more often affected; attacks last from 2 to 45 min and may occur up to 40 times per day. The syndrome responds to preventive treatment with indomethacin. SUNCT syndrome (shortlasting unilateral neuralgiform headache with conjunctival injection and tearing) targets mainly men; attacks have a duration of seconds to minutes and may occur up to 30 times per hour. The preventive treatment of choice is lamotrigine. Importantly, other conditions, including carotid artery dissection, tumors, and inflammatory infectious diseases, may mimic cluster headache (5). These so-called symptomatic cluster headache conditions exhibit red flags, i.e., late onset, prolonged attacks, and abnormal findings on neurological examination which must be further investigated. A cranial MRI with arteriogram and venogram sequences should be performed in these instances.

Treatment goals are twofold and include abortion of the individual attacks and shortening of the cluster period. Cluster headache attacks do not respond to standard analgesics. Inhalation of pure oxygen, flow rate of 7–10 l/min by a facial mask, provides relief in approximately 60% of cases. Attacks usually stop within 15 min (6, 7). There are no side-effects but the patient requires access to an oxygen supply. Before the availability of triptans, ergotamines were the most effective treatment. Most patients are currently pre-scribed sumatriptan or other triptans. Sumatriptan can be injected subcutaneously and leads to a pain-free state within 20 min in approximately 75% of patients. The contraindications to its use include cardiovas-cular and cerebrovascular disorders, and untreated arterial hypertension. Intranasal zolmitriptan can also provide relief (8), as do other orally ingested trip-tans. Pre-emptive use with triptans may prevent clus-ter attacks but the data have not been conclusive. The mainstay of treatment is prevention of further attacks. First-line drugs are glucocorticosteroids and verapamil. Open studies and case series confirm the clinically well-known efficacy of steroids such as pred-nisone or dexamethasone. Approximately 70–80% of all cluster headache patients respond to the standard dosage of 1 mg/kg of steroid. Patients typically experi-ence some relief of their symptoms within 3 days. The initial dose is maintained for 5–7 days, then depend-ing on the response, the steroid is slowly tapered over 2–3 weeks (9). If relapses occur during tapering, the steroid can be increased again or verapamil may be added. In some patients, a maintenance dose over the estimated time period of the cluster, i.e., 2 months, may be required. In refractory cases, pulse therapy with 500–1000 g of methylprednisolone for 3 days is rec-ommended. Verapamil is also efficient in reducing the cluster duration, although full efficacy may require 2–3 weeks of use. There is no consensus on a standard dose and the range of prescribed strengths is from 240 to 960 mg/day. An increase of 80 mg every 14 days is recommended. Regular echocardiographs are neces-sary to monitor the development of a prolonged PR interval (9). Further treatment options in refractory cases are topiramate and lithium, the latter in particu-lar in chronic cluster headache (10). In the more com-mon episodic type, it is important that the preventive treatment is tapered and discontinued when the clus-ter period has passed. For patients who do not respond satisfactorily to drug treatment, other options include suboccipital injection of steroids (11), occipital nerve stimulation (12), or even deep brain stimulation (13).

Pain in cluster headache

The typical attack has been described above. Attacks often occur when the patient is asleep. There is rapid onset of a headache that reaches its maximum inten-sity within 10 min and lasts for 30 to 180 min. The pain is almost always unilateral and rarely switches sides. The most common sites of maximal pain are the orbital, retro-orbital, temporal, supraorbital, and infraorbital areas. Cranial autonomic symptoms or the typical restlessness must be present to confirm the diagnosis. Patients usually experience 1 to 3 attacks per 24 h. Symptoms in cluster may be similar to those of migraine including nausea, photophobia, and phono-phobia (14).

Apart from the extreme pain intensity and patients' vivid descriptions of the attack, temporal periodicity is the most salient characteristic of cluster headache. Attacks often occur at the same time every night as the 2 am awakening described in this vignette. There may be a mirror-like, sometimes milder attack in the early afternoon. These attacks occur in clusters or bouts that may persist for weeks to months until the attacks become milder and eventually cease. Patients may be pain free for several months to years until the onset of the next cluster, a condition referred to as episodic cluster headache. Rarely, the attacks may persist for several years in which case the diagnosis is chronic cluster headache. The IHS defines this condition as the absence of remission for 1 year or by short remissions of less than 1 month.

A pathophysiological model for cluster headache must somehow account for the unilateral localization of the pain, the ipsilateral autonomic symptoms, the typical circadian occurrence of individual attacks, and the seasonal recurrence of the cluster periods (15). The proposal that pathology in the cavernous sinus such as inflammation is responsible for this condition has been recently challenged (16). Symptomatic clus-ter headache secondary to venous thrombosis or to other pathologies involving the cavernous sinus may be relevant considerations (17, 18). The severe unilat-eral pain is likely mediated by activation of the first division of the trigeminal nerve. Trigemino-vascular activation, as in the case of migraine, is considered the common final pathway of pain generation, supported by the rapid actions of triptans in the attacks.

Due to the intriguing temporal characteristics of the attacks, cluster headache has also been viewed as a disturbance of the biological clock caused by hypotha-lamic dysfunction. Hormonal alterations are described in men with cluster headache (19). Similarly, the auto-nomic symptoms are regarded as a consequence of hypothalamic disturbance with trigeminal discharge

(15). Parasympathetic hyperactivity with increased outflow from the seventh cranial nerve may lead to vasodilation and perivascular edema, which results in compression of sympathetic fibers around the carotid artery (20). The posterior hypothalamus is activated during an attack as demonstrated by positron emission tomography (PET) (21). This has also led to the use of hypothalamic stimulation as a treatment option in severe cases. In summary, most experts regard cluster headache as a syndrome involving peripheral and central pain generators. The pathophysiology may also involve deficits of pain inhibition or alterations in hypothalamic function.

References

(1) Horton BT, MacLean AR, Craig WM. A new syndrome of vascular headache; results of treatment with histamine: a preliminary report. *Mayo Clin Proc* 1939;14:250–257.

(2) Fischera M, Marziniak M, Gralow I, Evers S. The incidence and prevalence of cluster headache: a meta-analysis of population-based studies. *Cephalalgia* 2008;28:614–618.

(3) Lampl C. Childhood-onset cluster headache. *Pediatr Neurol* 2002;27:138–140.

(4) Sjostrand C, Russell MB, Ekbom K, Waldenlind E. Familial cluster headache: demographic patterns in affected and nonaffected. *Headache* 2010;50:374–382.

(5) Mainardi F, Trucco M, Maggioni F, Palestini C, Dainese F, Zanchin G. Cluster-like headache. A comprehensive reappraisal. *Cephalalgia* 2010;30:399–412.

(6) Fogan L. Treatment of cluster headache. A double-blind comparison of oxygen v air inhalation. *Arch Neurol* 1985;42:362–363.

(7) Cohen AS, Burns B, Goadsby PJ. High-flow oxygen for treatment of cluster headache: a randomized trial. *JAMA* 2009;302:2451–2457.

(8) Law S, Derry S, Moore RA. Triptans for acute cluster headache. *Cochrane Database Syst Rev* 2010:CD008042.

(9) May A, Leone M, Afra J, et al. EFNS guidelines on the treatment of cluster headache and other trigeminal-autonomic cephalalgias. *Eur J Neurol* 2006;13:1066–1077.

(10) Ashkenazi A, Schwedt T. Cluster headache–acute and prophylactic therapy. *Headache* 2011;51: 272–286.

(11) Leroux E, Valade D, Taifas I, et al. Suboccipital steroid injections for transitional treatment of patients with more than two cluster headache attacks per day: a randomised, double-blind, placebo-controlled trial. *Lancet Neurol* 2011;10:891–897.

(12) Magis D, Gerardy PY, Remacle JM, Schoenen J. Sustained effectiveness of occipital nerve stimulation in drug-resistant chronic cluster headache. *Headache* 2011;51:1191–1201.

(13) May A. Hypothalamic deep-brain stimulation: target and potential mechanism for the treatment of cluster headache. *Cephalalgia* 2008;28:799–803.

(14) Bahra A, Goadsby PJ. Diagnostic delays and mis-management in cluster headache. *Acta Neurol Scand* 2004;109:175–179.

(15) Leone M, Bussone G. Pathophysiology of trigeminal autonomic cephalalgias. *Lancet Neurol* 2009;8:755–764.

(16) Schuh-Hofer S, Richter M, Israel H, et al. The use of radiolabelled human serum albumin and SPECT/MRI co-registration to study inflammation in the cavernous sinus of cluster headache patients. *Cephalalgia* 2006;26:1115–1122.

(17) Park KI, Chu K, Park JM, Kim M. Cluster-like headache secondary to cerebral venous thrombosis. *J Clin Neurol* 2006;2:70–73.

(18) Palmieri A, Mainardi F, Maggioni F, Dainese F, Zanchin G. Cluster-like headache secondary to cavernous sinus metastasis. *Cephalalgia* 2005;25:743–745.

(19) May A. Cluster headache: pathogenesis, diagnosis, and management. *Lancet* 2005;366:843–855.

(20) Hardebo JE. How cluster headache is explained as an intracavernous inflammatory process lesioning sympathetic fibers. *Headache* 1994;34: 125–131.

(21) May A, Bahra A, Buchel C, Frackowiak RS, Goadsby PJ. Hypothalamic activation in cluster headache attacks. *Lancet* 1998;352:275–278.

(22) Headache Classification Subcommittee of the International Headache Society. The International Classification of Headache Disorders: 2nd edition. *Cephalalgia* 2004;24(Suppl 1):9–160.

29

Paroxysmal hemicrania

Paroxysmal hemicrania is a rare primary headache syndrome characterized by repeated attacks of strictly unilateral, severe, short-lasting pain associated with cranial autonomic symptoms. Recognition of the syndrome is important because it responds specifically to indomethacin.

Clinical case vignette

A 38-year-old woman presented with a 3-year history of facial pain. The pain was localized to the left upper jaw and radiated to the left temple and to the back of her head [Figure 29.1]. Pain attacks of 5- to 15-min duration were experienced at a rate of 10–20 per day. The severity of the attacks was such that the patient was forced to stop her activities. In the intervals between attacks, she was completely pain free. The patient had a long history of specialist consultations. She had first seen a dentist, whom she had instructed to extract a left upper molar, although the dentist was unconvinced of any existing pathology. The pain persisted despite the extraction. Her family physician diagnosed trigeminal neuralgia and performed acupuncture for 2 months without success. The patient then went to see a neurologist who diagnosed a "vascular facial pain," prescribing a sympathomimetic and a benzodiazepine. The drug combination reduced neither pain severity nor frequency of attacks. She then consulted a further neurological specialist in an outpatient clinic. The diagnosis was "atypical facial pain" and amitriptyline was prescribed. The patient tried using this drug in ascending doses up to 125 mg/day for 6 months with no success. Side-effects included dry mouth, constipation, and orthostatic hypotension. She stopped using amitriptyline and consulted a second dentist. This dentist diagnosed craniomandibular dysfunction, gave injections with a local anesthetic, and prescribed a splint. The patient wore the splint for 3 months but experienced no improvement. The dentist then advised the patient

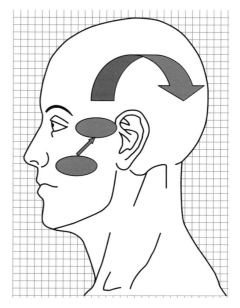

Figure 29.1. Reproduction of pain drawing based on the patient's original sketch.

to see an orthopedic surgeon. This specialist diagnosed neuralgia of the left occipitalis major and auricularis magnus nerve. He prescribed the analgesic flupirtine and additionally attempted chiropraxy to the temporomandibular joint. The outcome remained unsuccessful, and the patient next consulted an anesthesiological pain specialist from whom she received three diagnoses: atypical facial pain, cluster headache, and spondylosis of the cervical spine. Treatment was multimodal. For the first time in the course of her long history, the patient was advised to keep a pain diary. Pharmacological treatment with a combination of carbamazepine and doxepine was started. A local anesthetic was injected at regular intervals into trigger points of the cervical musculature. The patient further received lymph drainage, relaxation therapy, and conflict-centered psychotherapy. Several months later and still seeking relief, the patient consulted a further neurologist. This neurologist suspected pathology in the temporomandibular joint and referred the patient to an orthodontic surgeon. However, the patient decided to see a second anesthesiologist and visited a clinic specializing in radiofrequency therapy. Radiofrequency facet denervation was performed at several levels of the cervical spinal cord. With no therapeutic relief after several treatment sessions, the patient appeared at our Neurology outpatient clinic.

At the time of consultation, the patient was pain free. Neurologic and psychological examination were completely normal. There was no tenderness of pericranial or cervical muscles. Upon detailed history taking, the patient reported that sometimes during the pain attacks, her left eye became red and she noticed lacrimation. Based on the temporal characteristics of the pain attacks, the localization, and the associated symptoms, a diagnosis of chronic paroxysmal hemicrania was made. An initial dose of indomethacin 50 mg/day was prescribed with gradual increases to a maximum of 250 mg. The patient's attacks ceased entirely with a dose of 150 mg. Indomethacin was tapered to 12.5 mg/day, and the patient remained stable and tolerated the drug well.

Pain description

The patient gave a precise description of her pain. She described attacks of 10 to 15 min in duration. In the intervals between attacks, she was completely pain free. The pain was localized to the left upper jaw and radiated to the left temple and back of the head. It was strictly unilateral and never changed sides. The attacks occurred 10 to 20 times per day. During most attacks, the left eye became red with tears. There were no precipitating factors, and the onset of the attacks was unpredictable. Severity was gauged at 6–8/10, and there was very little if anything the patient could do to reduce pain severity. She sometimes took novamin sulfone drops and had the impression that these offered some relief. During the attacks, the patient stopped her activities when possible and waited for the attack to subside.

Discussion

PH is classified among the trigemino-autonomic cephalalgias (1). It is important to recognize trigemino autonomic headaches, and in particular PH, because patients often consult dentists or other oral health care

Table 29.1. IHS criteria of paroxysmal hemicrania (summarized from Headache Classification Committee (3))

Paroxysmal hemicrania	
Description	Attacks with similar characteristics of pain and associated symptoms and signs to those of cluster headache, but shorter-lasting, more frequent and commonly in females, that exclusively respond to indomethacin.
Diagnostic criteria:	A. At least 20 attacks fulfilling criteria B–D
	B. Attacks of severe unilateral orbital, supraorbital or temporal pain lasting 2–30 min
	C. Headache is accompanied by at least one of the following:
	1. ipsilateral conjunctival injection and/or lacrimation
	2. ipsilateral nasal congestion and/or rhinorrhoea
	3. ipsilateral eyelid oedema
	4. ipsilateral forehead and facial sweating
	5. ipsilateral miosis and/or ptosis
	D. Attacks have a greater frequency than 5 per day for more than 50% of the time, although periods with lower frequency may occur
	E. Attacks are completely prevented by therapeutic doses of indomethacin (at least 150 mg p.o. must be prescribed to confirm a response)
	F. Not attributed to another disorder

providers. There is a considerable risk that unnecessary, sometimes irreversible, procedures, i.e., tooth extraction, are attempted (2).

The term trigeminal autonomic cephalalgias refers to a group of headaches characterized by unilateral head or face pain with accompanying autonomic features. The International Headache Society's (IHS) criteria for PH are given in Table 29.1 (3). The hallmark feature of PH is cessation of the pain attacks upon treatment with indomethacin, a distinguishing feature that differentiates PH from the other trigemino-autonomic headaches. Episodic PH may be diagnosed if there are pain-free periods of one month or longer. In all other cases, the diagnosis is chronic paroxysmal hemicrania (CPH). PH was first described by Sjaastand and Dale as a new treatable headache entity in 1974 (4). PH is characterized by intense, strictly unilateral pain attacks localized to the temporal region, the orbita, the forehead or the ear, or a combination of those areas. The localization is similar to that in cluster headache. Associated symptoms, including ipsilateral conjunctival injection and lacrimation, are also described lasting 2–30 min (5) and are thus shorter than those of cluster headache, which last 30–90 min, and are considerably longer than those in SUNCT, another trigemino-autonomic cephalalgia (Short-lasting, Unilateral, Neuralgiform headache attacks with Conjunctival injection and Tearing), which last for mere seconds. Attacks are also more frequent than those experienced in cluster headache. The attacks typically last 10–15 min. While cluster headache usually occurs 1–2 times per 24 h, PH attacks may occur 10–20 times per day. Furthermore, more women than men suffer from PH while approximately 80% of cluster headache patients are men. During PH attacks, patients usually sit quietly or lie down in bed, activity that contrasts with that during cluster headache, where patients feel compelled to walk around (2). Attacks are more frequent during the day but may also occur during the night. Nighttime attacks are sometimes longer and more severe (6).

In addition to lacrimation and conjunctival injection, some patients have ipsilateral eyelid edema and miosis. Photophobia and phonophobia, often ipsilateral to the pain, may occur and may bring to mind the differential diagnosis of migraine, although individual migraine attacks are of much longer duration.

Pain in paroxysmal hemicrania

PH pain is unilateral and always affects the same side. Patients describe an excruciating, throbbing, boring, or pulsating pain. Triggers are observed by a minority of patients and may include exercise or stress (6). Between attacks, most patients are entirely pain free. Some have intermittent tenderness in the symptomatic area. In the presence of severe pain between attacks, the differential diagnosis of hemicrania continua must be considered (7). Hemicrania continua is described as persistent strictly unilateral headache responsive to indomethacin. As in PH, there are also autonomic symptoms but these are less consistent.

The exact prevalence of PH is not known but it is rare, attributing to the long delay between onset and diagnosis. PH was first reported in women only. Later studies found a female/male ratio of 2.4/1 (8) or even of 1/1 (6), although the latter contradicts the authors' clinical experience. The onset is usually in the third decade (mid-range) of adulthood. PH has also been reported in children (9).

The etiology and pathophysiology of PH are unknown. A primary CNS disorder with disturbance of the central control of sympathetic and parasympathetic systems is assumed. Some clue to a possible mechanism may lie in its exclusive response to indomethacin. Indomethacin, in contrast to other NSAIDS, reduces nitric oxide–induced dural vasodilation (10). Thus, the effect on prostaglandin synthesis may not be relevant for the treatment effect in PH because other NSAIDS are not effective in PH.

Cases of secondary PH with an underlying pathology (11) are possible. Among the differential diagnoses are intracranial tumors (12), collagenoses (13) and arteriovenous malformations (14). In patients with a poor response to indomethacin or with additional neurologic symptoms or signs, a brain MRI scan and blood tests for inflammation markers should be performed.

No agents have proven efficacious in aborting an acute PH attack. There is anecdotal evidence of some pain alleviation by sumatriptan (15) or by novamine sulfone. Standard treatment is prophylaxis with indomethacin. Drug doses should be initiated at 50 mg and increased to at least 150 mg/day for 3–4 days, with a maximum dose of 250 mg/day. Pain relief should occur within a few hours to days. The drug may then be tapered to a maintenance dose of between 25 to 100 mg/day although this varies between patients. Unfortunately when indomethacin is stopped, the headache returns. Common side-effects are gastritis, gastric ulcers, and bleeding, therefore, a gastric protective agent should be prescribed. If indomethacin cannot be tolerated, a COX-2 inhibitor (celecoxib) may be prescribed. A response to 150 mg/day of topiramate has also been described in some case reports (16, 17). Occipital nerve stimulation is another option for patients who are unresponsive to or cannot tolerate indomethacin (18). Deep brain stimulation has been suggested for patients who are unresponsive to other treatments (19).

References

(1) May A. Update on the diagnosis and management of trigemino-autonomic headaches. *J Neurol* 2006;253:1525–1532.

(2) Klasser GD, Balasubramaniam R. Trigeminal autonomic cephalalgias. Part 2: Paroxysmal hemicrania. *Oral Surg Oral Med Oral Pathol Oral Radiol Endod* 2007;104:640–646.

(3) Headache Classification Committee of the International Headache Society. The International Classification of Headache Disorders. 2nd edition. *Cephalalgia* 2004;24(Suppl 1):1–160.

(4) Sjaastad O, Dale I. Evidence for a new (?), treatable headache entity. *Headache* 1974;14:105–108.

(5) Russell D. Chronic paroxysmal hemicrania: severity, duration and time of occurrence of attacks. *Cephalalgia* 1984;4:53–56.

(6) Cittadini E, Matharu MS, Goadsby PJ. Paroxysmal hemicrania: a prospective clinical study of 31 cases. *Brain* 2008;131:1142–1155.

(7) Goadsby PJ, Cittadini E, Cohen AS. Trigeminal autonomic cephalalgias: paroxysmal hemicrania, SUNCT/SUNA, and hemicrania continua. *Semin Neurol* 2010;30:186–191.

(8) Sjaastad O, Bakketeig LS. The rare, unilateral headaches. Vaga study of headache epidemiology. *J Headache Pain* 2007;8:19–27.

(9) Blankenburg M, Hechler T, Dubbel G, Wamsler C, Zernikow B. Paroxysmal hemicrania in children – symptoms, diagnostic criteria, therapy and outcome. *Cephalalgia* 2009;29:873–882.

(10) Summ O, Andreou AP, Akerman S, Goadsby PJ. A potential nitrergic mechanism of action for indomethacin, but not of other COX inhibitors: relevance to indomethacin-sensitive headaches. *J Headache Pain* 2010;11:477–483.

(11) Trucco M, Mainardi F, Maggioni F, Badino R, Zanchin G. Chronic paroxysmal hemicrania, hemicrania continua and SUNCT syndrome in association with other pathologies: a review. *Cephalalgia* 2004;24:173–184.

(12) Dafer RM, Hocker S, Kumar R, McGee J, Jay WM. Resolution of paroxysmal hemicrania after resection of intracranial meningioma. *Semin Ophthalmol* 2010;25:34–35.

(13) Medina JL. Organic headaches mimicking chronic paroxysmal hemicrania. *Headache* 1992;32:73–74.

(14) Newman LC, Herskovitz S, Lipton RB, Solomon S. Chronic paroxysmal headache: two cases with cerebrovascular disease. *Headache* 1992;32: 75–76.

(15) Pascual J, Quijano J. A case of chronic paroxysmal hemicrania responding to subcutaneous sumatriptan. *J Neurol Neurosurg Psychiatry* 1998;65:407.

(16) Cohen AS, Goadsby PJ. Paroxysmal hemicrania responding to topiramate. *J Neurol Neurosurg Psychiatry* 2007;78:96–97.

(17) Camarda C, Camarda R, Monastero R. Chronic paroxysmal hemicrania and hemicrania continua responding to topiramate: two case reports. *Clin Neurol Neurosurg* 2008;110:88–91.

(18) Burns B, Watkins L, Goadsby PJ. Treatment of hemicrania continua by occipital nerve stimulation with a bion device: long-term follow-up of a crossover study. *Lancet Neurol* 2008;7:1001–1012.

(19) Franzini A, Messina G, Cordella R, Marras C, Broggi G. Deep brain stimulation of the posteromedial hypothalamus: indications, long-term results, and neurophysiological considerations. *Neurosurg Focus* 2010;29:E13.

Trigeminal neuralgia

Trigeminal neuralgia is a very characteristic facial pain of the elderly, and is usually caused by neurovascular compression adjacent in the brainstem. In this older age group, it is important that the diagnosis of trigeminal neuralgia be differentiated from trigeminal neuropathy. If it occurs in a young patient, investigations into an underlying disorder must be considered.

Clinical case vignette

A 75-year-old male presented with an 8-week history of severe pain attacks in the area of the left upper jaw. He had experienced a similar episode approximately 12 months previously but the pain had spontaneously resolved after 6 weeks. The individual attacks only lasted for a few seconds, but they were extremely severe and could occur frequently on a daily basis. During the last 2 weeks, the pain had progressively intensified and the number of attacks had increased. The attacks were usually precipitated by the patient washing his face, brushing his teeth, shaving, eating, and talking. To avoid the onset of new attacks, he refused to eat and drink. His wife became worried and convinced him to see a doctor. On examination, the patient was dehydrated, mildly slowed, but fully oriented. He refused to have his left face touched and spoke minimally, indicating to his wife to speak for him. His neurological examination was otherwise normal. A diagnosis of trigeminal neuralgia involving its second branch, the maxillary nerve, was made. The patient was admitted to the ward, and given intravenous fluids and a long-acting opioid with rapid onset. After an EKG confirmed the absence of heart block, 250 mg of intravenous phenytoin was slowly administered followed by 100 mg of oral phenytoin tid. Carbamazepine was started at a dose of 200 mg bid, and increased to 400 mg bid over the next 2 days at which time the phenytoin was tapered. The patient reported relief of pain almost immediately after the infusion and experienced very few attacks with full doses of carbamazepine. Despite

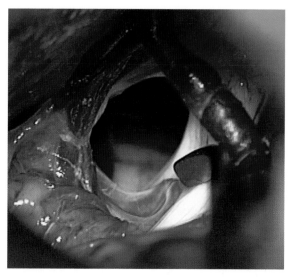

Figure 30.1. Intraoperative photograph showing the trigeminal nerve (TN) and the superior cerebellar artery, which is compressing the nerve. The neurosurgeon is mobilizing the artery with a small spatula. Courtesy Dr. José Perez, Department of Neurosurgery, University Würzburg, Germany.

ongoing treatment, the patient experienced a return of his pain 6 months later. The dose of carbamazepine was increased to 600 mg bid but the resulting side-effects of dizziness and unsteady gait were intolerable. Cranial MRI showed contact between the trigeminal nerve and a vascular loop. After a neurosurgical consultation, a Janetta nerve decompression operation was successfully performed [Figure 30.1]. At his 2-year follow-up visit, the patient continued to experience full remission.

Pain description

The patient described the pain attacks as stabbing and electric-shock–like. The pain was felt in the skin and deep tissues in the area of the left lower face and radiated to the corner of the mouth [Figure 30.2]. These very brief attacks sometimes came in episodes lasting

Table 30.1. International Headache Society (IHS) diagnostic criteria of trigeminal neuralgia (1)

Paroxysmal attacks of pain lasting from a fraction of a second to 2 min, affecting one or more divisions of the trigeminal nerve and
Pain has at least one of the following characteristics:
1. intense, sharp, superficial or stabbing
2. precipitated from trigger areas or by trigger factors
Attacks are stereotyped in the individual patient
There is no clinically evident neurological deficit
The pain cannot be attributed to another disorder

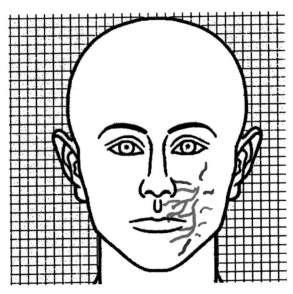

Figure 30.2. Pain drawing by the patient. The area of most severe, stabbing pain is depicted in red.

up to 10 min. Afterward, there was a short period during which the patient was pain free, even if he touched his facial skin. Otherwise, pain attacks could be induced by touching the skin, talking, eating, brushing the teeth, and shaving. The patient consequently avoided these activities as much as possible. Standard analgesics (acetaminophen, aspirin) neither reduced the pain nor diminished the number of attacks.

Discussion

Trigeminal neuralgia is characterized by brief attacks of unilateral pain in the territory of one or more branches of the trigeminal nerve; the diagnostic criteria for this condition, as defined by the International Headache Society (IHS), are listed in Table 30.1 (1). It has an overall prevalence of 1:30000 and occurs mostly in elderly patients, more often in women than in men. Younger patients with trigeminal neuralgia likely have an additional underlying disease; see below.

The pathogenesis of what is now called "typical" trigeminal neuralgia was initially suspected by the neurosurgeon Dandy approximately 80 years ago (see Prasad and Galetta (2)). Compression of the trigeminal nerve at the entry zone into the pons was later confirmed to be present in 80–90% of patients with typical trigeminal neuralgia. The superior cerebellar artery is usually involved. In the trigeminal nerve root, fibers of the second trigeminal branch, V2, are located medially. Because compression typically occurs at this point, pain in the distribution of the maxillary nerve is the most common manifestation of typical trigeminal neuralgia. An MRI scan, using specific sequences, can confirm the compression of the nerve by a vascular loop with a sensitivity of almost 100% (3, 4) (Figure 30.1). Specificity is lower, because a neurovascular contact can also be found in approximately 50% on the contralateral side (5) and in up to 20% of asymptomatic controls; this finding is only relevant in the presence of clinical symptoms.

The pathological process is assumed to mainly occur in the transition zone between central myelin and peripheral myelin at the entry zone of the trigeminal root into the pons. CNS myelin, synthesized by oligodendrocytes, is more vulnerable to compression than peripheral nerve myelin. Focal demyelination, close to the vascular indentation, has been observed (6). Thinly myelinated A-delta nociceptive fibers seem particularly vulnerable to these changes. The demyelination leads to direct membrane-to-membrane contact of axons, to spontaneous activity, and to mechanosensitization from pressure by the overlying artery. Ephaptic impulse propagation between fibers mediating tactile impulses and nociceptors is a possible explanation for the triggering of pain sensations. Furthermore, partially injured sensory neurons may develop bursts of "after discharge." This means that discharges extend beyond the duration of a stimulus. Neighboring neurons may be recruited, which leads to a further increase of the electrical activity and thus of the pain. The electrical activity is terminated by hyperpolarization due to the influx of potassium ions (7).

When the compression is relieved operatively, pain usually ceases immediately. This is explained by the reduction in ectopic impulse generation (6). Progressive demyelination may also be associated with axonal damage, such that trigeminal neuralgia can induce spontaneous continuous pain in the long-term or on a chronic basis. At this stage, the success rate of neurovascular decompression is considerably reduced (8).

Young patients in an age range of 15–45 years who are afflicted with trigeminal neuralgia must be investigated for an underlying disease. Multiple sclerosis presents with symptoms resembling trigeminal neuralgia in 1–5% of cases. Other symptomatic causes include tumors of the cerebellar pontine angle, aneurysms, or ischemic brain infarction. In these conditions, a cranial MRI scan can exclude a tumor, an aneurysm, a cerebral infarct, or an inflammatory demyelinating lesion diagnostic of multiple sclerosis. Neurophysiologic tests including the blink reflex, the masseter reflex, and evoked potentials of the trigeminal nerve may also substantiate a trigeminal nerve lesion. If multiple sclerosis is suspected, cerebrospinal fluid and neurophysiologic investigation are helpful.

Because the pain attacks or sensations induced by trigeminal neuralgia are brief, medical treatment is best directed toward reducing the number of attacks. Drugs acting at voltage-gated sodium channels appear most therapeutic. Carbamazepine remains the drug of choice and is the only drug tested in several placebo-controlled randomized controlled trials. The therapeutic dose is between 800 and 1600 mg/day; the initial dose of 200 mg bid should be gradually and carefully incremented. Sustained-release formulations are preferable. The initial response rate to carbamazepine is almost 90%. Increases in dosage strength may be necessary throughout the duration of the disease. Side-effects include sedation, dizziness, and unsteady gait; these issues must be addressed while achieving a therapeutic dose. If rapid onset of action is needed, phenytoin can be given intravenously (off label use) at 250 mg bid after exclusion of conduction block by EKG, or orally using 100 mg tid. Second-line drugs are lamotrigine, which has been used as an add-on medication in one small trial, and gabapentin, which has been efficient in open-label trials. Case reports describe successful pain control with valproic acid, oxcarbazepine, pregabalin, and topiramate; data from randomized controlled trials are unavailable. Misoprostol was useful in a small case series of patients with multiple sclerosis.

Spontaneous remissions may occur in the natural history of trigeminal neuralgia. The weaning of pain medication may be considered in a patient who has been asymptomatic for at least 2 months. If symptoms recur, the same drug may be used again and is likely to be therapeutic for a second course.

Interventional treatment procedures may be indicated if drug therapy is unsuccessful (9). These include microvascular decompression in the cerebello-pontine angle, percutaneous procedures at the Gasserian ganglion, and radiosurgical treatment. Based on the pathomechanism of neurovascular compression, the surgical procedure named after Janetta (10) may successfully abolish the underlying cause of trigeminal neuralgia. Healthy patients capable of undergoing general anesthesia are eligible. The trigeminal root is decompressed by a retrosigmoidal approach through the occipital fossa, the trigeminal root is identified, and if a compressing artery can be seen, it is separated from the nerve (Figure 30.2). Short- and long-term success rates are good with acute improvement in 87–98% of patients and long-term results at 8 years in 60% of patients. The rate of complications is 1–2% with rare serious complications (2, 11).

Older patients in poor general health can be treated with selective percutaneous high frequency thermolesions of the Gasserian ganglion. Under radiographic control, a needle is introduced into the foramen ovale. Radiofrequency stimulation is used to selectively destroy the nociceptive trigeminal fibers. The relapse rate is 20% in 10 years but the procedure can be repeated. This method can also be helpful in patients with multiple sclerosis. Percutaneous balloon compression is an alternate procedure (12). Because both are essentially destructive procedures, numbness and dysesthesias may occur as side-effects, more rarely keratitis, anesthesia dolorosa, and dysfunction of masticatory muscles. Stereotactic gamma knife radiosurgery is a third procedure considerably less destructive than the above. It has an initial success rate of 86% and 75% at 33 months (13). Complications are mild and occur in approximately 10% of cases. This method has shown efficacy in patients with trigeminal neuralgia caused by multiple sclerosis (14).

Pain in trigeminal neuralgia

The pain attacks in trigeminal neuralgia are typically described as lancinating, stabbing, or electric-shock–like. They may occur spontaneously or be triggered by trivial stimuli such as touching the skin, chewing, talking, brushing the teeth, shaving, or even a breeze of air. The second or third branch of the trigeminal nerve is most commonly involved. An individual attack may last a mere second but because they usually occur in clusters, patients may report that they last for longer durations of time. Fearing the onset of new attacks, elderly patients may avoid fluid and food intake, and may present in the clinic in a dehydrated, often confused state. Some patients become suicidal. The pathophysiology is assumed to entail demyelination of nociceptive A-delta fibers at the entrance into the pons. This is believed to lead to a faster spread of excitation, for example through ephaptic connections between nerve fibers. The explanation is plausible considering the therapeutic actions of the sodium channel blocker carbamazepine in this disease.

References

(1) Headache Classification Committee of the International Headache Society. The International Classification of Headache Disorders. 2nd edition. *Cephalalgia* 2004;24(Suppl 1):1–160.

(2) Prasad S, Galetta S. Trigeminal neuralgia: historical notes and current concepts. *Neurologist* 2009;15: 87–94.

(3) Meaney JF, Eldridge PR, Dunn LT, Nixon TE, Whitehouse GH, Miles JB. Demonstration of neurovascular compression in trigeminal neuralgia with magnetic resonance imaging. Comparison with surgical findings in 52 consecutive operative cases. *J Neurosurg* 1995;83:799–805.

(4) Patel A, Kassam A, Horowitz M, Chang YF. Microvascular decompression in the management of glossopharyngeal neuralgia: analysis of 217 cases. *Neurosurgery* 2002;50:705–710; discussion 710–711.

(5) Lorenzoni J, David P, Devriendt D. Patterns of neurovascular compression in patients with classic trigeminal neuralgia: a high-resolution MRI-based study. *Eur J Radiol* 2009 [Epub ahead of print].

(6) Love S, Coakham HB. Trigeminal neuralgia: pathology and pathogenesis. *Brain* 2001;124: 2347–2360.

(7) Zakrzewska JM, McMillan R. Trigeminal neuralgia: the diagnosis and management of this excruciating and poorly understood facial pain. *Postgrad Med J* 2011;87:410–416.

(8) Tyler-Kabara EC, Kassam AB, Horowitz MH, et al. Predictors of outcome in surgically managed patients with typical and atypical trigeminal neuralgia: comparison of results following microvascular decompression. *J Neurosurg* 2002;96:527–531.

(9) Zakrzewska JM, Akram H. Neurosurgical interventions for the treatment of classical trigeminal neuralgia. *Cochrane Database Syst Rev* 2011;9: CD007312.

(10) Jannetta PJ. Outcome after microvascular decompression for typical trigeminal neuralgia, hemifacial spasm, tinnitus, disabling positional vertigo, and glossopharyngeal neuralgia (honored guest lecture). *Clin Neurosurg* 1997;44:331–383.

(11) Sekula RF, Marchan EM, Fletcher LH, Casey KF, Jannetta PJ. Microvascular decompression for trigeminal neuralgia in elderly patients. *J Neurosurg* 2008;108:689–691.

(12) Skirving DJ, Dan NG. A 20-year review of percutaneous balloon compression of the trigeminal ganglion. *J Neurosurg* 2001;94:913–917.

(13) Kondziolka D, Lunsford LD, Flickinger JC. Stereotactic radiosurgery for the treatment of trigeminal neuralgia. *Clin J Pain* 2002;18: 42–47.

(14) Regis J, Metellus P, Hayashi M, Roussel P, Donnet A, Bille-Turc F. Prospective controlled trial of gamma knife surgery for essential trigeminal neuralgia. *J Neurosurg* 2006;104:913–924.

Chapter 31

Headache and acute cerebral ischemia

Patients with an acute headache are often fearful of having experienced a stroke. When presented with cases of acute and severe headache however, neurologists are inclined to consider subarachnoid hemorrhage as the classic emergency diagnosis, requiring immediate action. Cerebral ischemia is less often considered in the context of acute headache. Headache at the onset of cerebral ischemia associated with stroke is illustrated in the following case study.

Clinical case vignette

A 24-year-old law student experienced a sudden attack of vertigo on a Sunday while at rest, without any prior exertion. Soon afterward, he noticed a headache that began at the back of his skull and gradually increased in intensity. On Monday, the headache intensity increased yet again, and the patient saw his general practitioner. Due to the severity of the headache in a young man who did not usually suffer from head pains, a diagnosis of subarachnoid hemorrhage was suspected. The patient was referred to the hospital emergency department that same night. He was found to have mild neck stiffness (meningismus), but was awake, alert, and had an otherwise normal neurological examination. An emergency cranial computed tomography (CT) did not detect intracranial blood and was considered normal. A spinal tap was performed in the expectation of finding hemorrhagic cerebrospinal fluid (CSF), confirming a diagnosis of subarachnoid hemorrhage. The CSF however, was clear and contained 50 cells/μl of mostly lymphocytes. A putative diagnosis of viral meningitis was made and CSF samples were sent for analysis. The patient received intravenous paracetamol for symptomatic treatment and headache intensity decreased from 6/10 to 3/10. The CT was re-evaluated, and a right cerebellar infarct was diagnosed [Figure 31.1a]. Magnetic resonance imaging (MRI) confirmed a large

infarct of the right posterior inferior cerebellar artery [Figure 31.1b]. The patient meanwhile had only mild headache, increased vertigo, and no other neurological symptoms or signs for the next 2 days. On the third day however, he awoke with nausea and vomited, and his headache again increased in severity. On examination, he had developed nystagmus on left gaze but no other neurological deficits. Head CT revealed swelling of the infarct with compression of the 4th ventricle, lateral shift of the 3rd ventricle, and visible lower horns of the lateral ventricles, indicating increased intracranial pressure due to edema in the peri-infarct area [Figure 31.1c]. The patient was transferred to the intensive care unit. A posterior fossa craniectomy was considered but postponed because the patient remained stable. He received osmotherapy and was closely monitored. Two days later, both the headache and nystagmus had resolved, and a control CT revealed normalization of the ventricles [Figure 31.1d]. The patient was subsequently discharged from the intensive care unit and investigated for a potential embolus that may have caused the stroke. Doppler sonography, 24-h EKG, laboratory tests for a coagulation disorder, and cerebral angiography were all normal. Finally, transesophageal echocardiography detected a patent foramen ovale with a hypermobile atrial septum. Anticoagulation with warfarin was considered the treatment of choice but was initiated only 2 weeks later to reduce the risk of hemorrhagic transformation of the infarct.

Pain description

The patient described a novel posterior headache that developed subacutely at the time of presentation then worsened on day 3, coincident with evidence for cerebellar edema. It was associated with nausea, vomiting, neck stiffness, and other symptoms and signs of cerebral ischemia. While the association has been

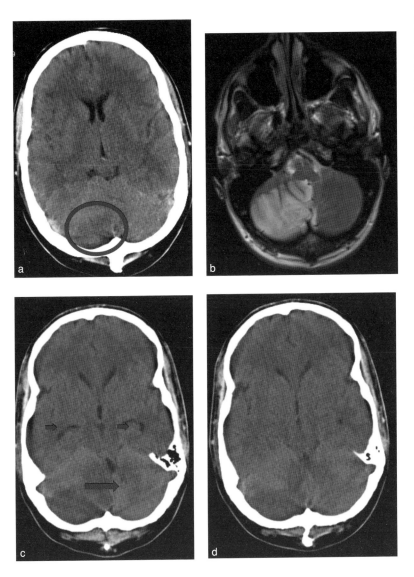

Figure 31.1. Cranial images from the patient presented in this vignette. A head CT scan in (a) showed mild hypointensity of the right cerebellum (circled), identified as an extensive infarction on a FLAIR sequence MR (b). Later on day 3 during his hospitalization, significant edema of the right cerebellar hemisphere with shift (large arrow) was identified with enlargement of the temporal horns of the lateral ventricles (small arrows). Two days later the ventricular enlargement had resolved, along with the headache (d). Courtesy of Prof. Solymosi, Department of Neuroradiology, University Hospital of Würzburg.

previously recognized, presentation of stroke with a new onset headache in a young patient is unusual.

Discussion

Two aspects of this case history are important: 1. The occurrence of headache at the onset of stroke without accompanying neurological deficits. 2. The renewed increase in headache intensity concurrent with the rise in intracranial pressure.

Upon initial presentation, our patient underwent a CT scan to rule out a subarachnoid bleed. Because CT is typically negative in the first hours after acute ischemic stroke and also has a low sensitivity for detecting early infarction in the posterior fossa, an MRI with diffusion-weighted imaging (DWI) is generally accepted as the investigation of choice (1). It must be noted however, that MRI also has low sensitivity in the cerebellum. While the overall sensitivity of DWI is 80–95% in the first 24 h, false-negative studies may occur, especially in the posterior circulation (2).

Our patient had no obvious risk factors. Risk factors for cerebellar infarcts are generally identical to those for ischemic stroke and include: hypertension, diabetes, cigarette smoking, hyperlipidaemia, and atrial fibrillation. Vertebral artery dissection after preceding trauma might have induced his stroke but a dissection was not visualized using duplex sonography or MRI. The patient had no history of trauma; however, a history of major or minor head or neck trauma, including chiropractic manipulations, is identified in fewer than half of cases of dissection (3). Patent foramen ovale is yet another potential cause of embolism in young patients. In a study involving patients younger than 40 years of age who suffered a cerebellar stroke, approximately 50% were found to have a patent foramen ovale (4). Less common causes include hypercoagulable states, vasculitis, and acute marijuana or cocaine use. In our patient, the presence of a patent foramen ovale with a hypermobile atrial septum was confirmed and the likely cause of his cerebellar stroke.

In our patient, the presence of a patent foramen ovale with a hypermobile atrial septum was confirmed and the likely cause of his cerebellar stroke.

Infarcts of the cerebellum often result in general symptoms including dizziness, nausea, vomiting, unsteady gait, and headache, all of which can be caused by common and benign disorders. Neurological signs, like dysarthria, ataxia, and nystagmus, may be absent or very mild (3). Of the three vascular areas in the cerebellum, the posterior inferior cerebellar artery (PICA), anterior inferior cerebellar artery (AICA), and superior cerebellar artery (SCA), the PICA appears most associated with headache and vertigo (5).

In our patient, the finding of CSF pleocytosis with 50 cells/μl could have been diagnostic of a viral meningitis. He had no fever and general malaise, which can also be typical of this condition. Furthermore, enteroviruses are known to cause syndromes with headache and gastrointestinal disturbance. Cerebral vasculitis, which can also cause stroke associated with headache, was considered but angiography of the cerebral arteries was normal. CSF analysis is not useful or even recommended in patients with stroke (and is contraindicated if a cerebellar stroke with swelling is suspected); there may be CSF pleocytosis of up to 60 cells/μl if a spinal tap is performed early in cerebral ischemia, particularly if the infarct is close to the subarachnoid surface (6).

The secondary increase in headache intensity associated with vomiting on day 4 of our patient's admission was likely due to increased intracranial pressure. Infarcts in the posterior fossa lead to edema formation resulting in compression of adjacent tissue in approximately 10–20% of patients. On average, edema peaks on the third day post-infarction but can occur at any time within the first 7 days (3). Approximately 50% of patients with radiographical evidence of a mass effect also deteriorate clinically due to increased intracranial pressure. They may experience double vision, disturbances of pupillary reaction and a progressive decline in level of consciousness. Corticosteroids have no effect and osmotic diuretics have only transient benefits. If craniectomy is attempted on patients who become comatose, the outcome is favorable in 50% of cases. Without surgery, there is an 85% risk of death (3).

Surgical intervention remains contentious. External ventricular drainage is considered the first measure. Suboccipital craniectomy with removal of the infarcted tissue is usually attempted next because craniectomy in itself carries an increased risk of morbidity and mortality (3).

Pain in acute cerebral ischemia

Headache is not usually considered a hallmark of ischemic stroke; the frequency of headache is higher in intracerebral hemorrhage than in ischemia (7, 8). However, headache at the onset of cerebral ischemia may occur and its frequency, characteristics, and relation to stroke localization are well documented (9). The incidence of headache is slightly higher in strokes of the posterior than the anterior circulation (15–65 vs. 8–46%). Also, headache intensity tends to be higher in posterior circulation ischemia. On average, 40% of patients with cerebellar stroke experience headache (10). Because patients typically manifest neurological deficits like hemiparesis or aphasia during an ischemic attack, headache is infrequently described. Physicians may fail to question patients regarding the presence of headache while patients may either be too anxious about their other neurological deficits or incapable of expressing themselves. This case, which highlights the constellation of headache as essentially the singular symptom in a large ischemic stroke, is striking. Data for this scenario are currently unavailable. It should be noted that headache may also be a symptom of a transient ischemic attack (TIA); several prospective studies suggest that this occurs in 16 to 36 of cases (11, 12). The frequency of headache in cardioembolic stroke is not different from that in large vessel disease. One exception however, may occur in the case of lacunar stroke where headache frequency is low, i.e., 1–23% (9). Headache quality in stroke does not appear to have any defining features and may mimic tension-type headache, migraine, or others. The pain is often pressure-like, or sometimes pulsating. Patients have also described stabbing or burning sensations. The localization of the pain is not strictly related to the site of the ischemia. Prospective studies have been unable to confirm past observations that patients with ischemia in the territory of the basilar artery may experience a severe throbbing occipital headache that is aggravated by stooping and straining (see Evans and Mitsias (9)). Similarly, the headache site is not helpful in predicting stroke localization. The onset of the headache may be acute or gradually increase in severity. The severity is greatest at presentation. A headache that is considered to be stroke-related must persist for a minimum of one day. The mean duration is 3.8 days. As with subarachnoid hemorrhage, a sentinel headache which occurs hours to days before the ischemic event may occur in approximately 10–43% of patients (13, 14).

Because headache is a common occurrence, it may be difficult to decide which patients require further investigations. Young patients with a headache associated with dizziness or vertigo should be monitored because these symptoms may be warning signs of cerebellar infarction or vertebral artery dissection (14). Most guidelines concur that physicians should be vigilant about and investigate all patients with new, abrupt-onset, persistent, or unusual headaches, particularly if located posteriorly or in the neck (15, 16). "Thunderclap" headaches may similarly herald cerebellar infarction (17).

The pathophysiology of stroke-related headache is unclear. Because there are no nociceptors in the brain parenchyma, pain signals come from meningeal afferents and the innervation of the large cerebral arteries. These are likely activated by stretching due to the edema associated with large infarcts. In cases of small to medium infarcts, other mechanisms of headache generation are presumed. These include direct ischemia of these structures or the release of algogenic substances, for example vasoactive neuropeptides or nitric oxide, from vessels related to the ischemic area (9). Stimulation of the trigeminovascular system by large vessel afferent fibers around the large arteries is assumed to be the final pathway. The density of perivascular innervation may be higher in the posterior circulation, a likely explanation for the higher prevalence of headache in this area.

The average age of patients diagnosed with cerebellar infarct is 65 years (3). This occurrence in our young patient is unusual. He had no family history of neurological disease. His complaints of vertigo and headache were initially diagnosed as a possible gastrointestinal disorder although vestibular migraine might have been a second possibility on his differential diagnosis. Vestibular migraine presents at any age and is known to peak in men in their fourth decade. It is characterized by repeated attacks of vertigo lasting seconds to hours and rarely days, as well as a mild to moderate headache.

In summary, occipital headache with vertigo may be indicative of cerebellar infarct. A secondary increase in headache character in a patient with cerebellar infarct is highly suspicious of increased intracranial pressure.

References

(1) Olivot JM, Albers GW. Diffusion-perfusion MRI for triaging transient ischemic attack and acute cerebrovascular syndromes. *Curr Opin Neurol* 2011;24:44–49.

(2) Oppenheim C, Stanescu R, Dormont D, et al. False-negative diffusion-weighted MR findings in acute ischemic stroke. *AJNR Am J Neuroradiol* 2000;21:1434–1440.

(3) Edlow JA, Newman-Toker DE, Savitz SI. Diagnosis and initial management of cerebellar infarction. *Lancet Neurol* 2008;7:951–964.

(4) Barinagarrementeria F, Amaya LE, Cantu C. Causes and mechanisms of cerebellar infarction in young patients. *Stroke* 1997;28:2400–2404.

(5) Kase CS, Norrving B, Levine SR, et al. Cerebellar infarction. Clinical and anatomic observations in 66 cases. *Stroke* 1993;24:76–83.

(6) Carhuapoma JR, Welch KMA. Cerebral spinal fluid in stroke. In: Welch KMA, Caplan LR, Reis DJ, Siesjö BK, Weir B, eds. *Primer on Cerebrovascular Diseases.* San Diego: Academic Press, 1997:597–599.

(7) Vestergaard K, Andersen G, Nielsen MI, Jensen TS. Headache in stroke. *Stroke* 1993;24:1621–1624.

(8) Jorgensen HS, Jespersen HF, Nakayama H, Raaschou HO, Olsen TS. Headache in stroke: the Copenhagen Stroke Study. *Neurology* 1994;44:1793–1797.

(9) Evans RW, Mitsias PD. Headache at onset of acute cerebral ischemia. *Headache* 2009;49:902–908.

(10) Tentschert S, Wimmer R, Greisenegger S, Lang W, Lalouschek W. Headache at stroke onset in 2196 patients with ischemic stroke or transient ischemic attack. *Stroke* 2005;36:e1–e3.

(11) Edmeads J. The headache of ischemic cerebrovascular disease. *Headache* 1979;19:345–349.

(12) Ferro JM, Costa I, Melo TP, et al. Headache associated with transient ischemic attacks. *Headache* 1995;35:544–548.

(13) Gorelick PB, Hier DB, Caplan LR, Langenberg P. Headache in acute cerebrovascular disease. *Neurology* 1986;36:1445–1450.

(14) Williams D, Wilson TG. The diagnosis of the major and minor syndromes of basilar insufficiency. *Brain* 1962;85:741–774.

(15) Jordan JE. Headache. *AJNR Am J Neuroradiol* 2007;28:1824–1826.

(16) Kim BM, Kim SH, Kim DI, et al. Outcomes and prognostic factors of intracranial unruptured vertebrobasilar artery dissection. *Neurology* 2011;76:1735–1741.

(17) Sutton Brown M, Morrish W, Zochodne DW. Recurrent coital "Thunderclap" headache associated with ischaemic stroke. *Cephalalgia* 2006;26:1028–1030.

Therapeutics in neuropathic pain

32

The specific mechanisms responsible for generating neuropathic pain continue to be unravelled. The hope is that novel and targeted approaches will offer better efficacy than current approaches. At the time of writing, these approaches are well dissected by guidelines and literature reviews, some recently published. None of the agents highlighted by these publications have offered dramatic pain relief and all therapeutic regimens suffer from potential side-effects. The guidelines and agents described in this chapter, therefore, are likely to be outdated soon as newer trials are completed and published. It is also important to emphasize that the recommendations, dosing schedules, and potential side-effects are only summarized here. They do not substitute for a detailed appraisal of proposed therapy in a given patient, and it is imperative for the clinician to consult primary literature and detailed drug monographs when considering therapy.

Overall considerations

Therapy for neuropathic pain should begin with consideration of nonpharmacological approaches such as the use of comfortable, properly fitting footware, treatment of associated foot ulcers, exclusion of other causes of pain, and simple self-limited use of analgesics. If possible, reversal of the underlying neurological cause for pain should be undertaken, a direction that may obviate the need for ongoing specific pain therapy. In many chronic neurological disorders with irreversible disability and damage however, this option is not available. Treatment needs to take into account the needs and preferences of patients and patients should have the opportunity to make informed decisions. Good communication is essential and should be supported by evidence-based written information. This material should also be culturally appropriate.

Overall approaches are to exclude other causes of pain, as well as evaluating and treating concurrent depression, underlying medical disorders (uncontrolled glycemic control in diabetes, hypertension, obesity, hyperlipidemia, smoking), and adjacent soft tissue injury, including ulcers. For allodynia, use of a blanket cradle to lift bedclothes from the feet is helpful. Abnormalities of gait may predispose patients to pain from hip, knee, and ankle injury. Some patients with more severe lower limb weakness may develop carpal tunnel syndrome from overuse of the upper limbs.

For pharmacological pain therapy, the major classes of agents used are antidepressants, including serotonin and norepinephrine uptake inhibitors, anti-epileptics ("anti-convulsants"), and opioids. Published guidelines also include other pharmacological approaches but uniformly admit that their evidence basis is lower tiered.

Guidelines

EFNS guidelines 2010 (1)

The most recent 2010 version of the EFNS guidelines for the treatment of neuropathic pain used a search of the Cochrane library from 2005 expanded to MEDLINE and other electronic databases including unpublished industry trials. Sixty-four RCTs (randomized controlled trials) using placebo or active drug comparators were identified. Level A evidence was presented for: duloxetine, gabapentin-morphine, tricylcic antidepressants, gabapentin, oxycodone, pregabalin, tramadol, and venlafaxine ER. Level B ratings for efficacy were described for botulinum toxin, dextromethorphan, gabapentin/venlafaxine, and levodopa. Carbamazepine and phenytoin achieved level C ratings for efficacy overall but carbamazepine had a specific level A rating in trigeminal neuralgia.

Recommendations were duloxetine, gabapentin, pregabalin, tricyclic antidepressants, and venlafaxine ER as first-line therapy and opioids, including tramadol, as second or third line.

Recommendations of IASP (International Association for the Study of Pain), NEUPSIG (Neuropathic Pain Special Interest Group)(2) 2010

This working group suggested symptomatic treatment of neuropathic pain with one of the following: 1. nortriptyline, desipramine, or an SNRI (serotonin and norepinephrine reuptake inhibitors specifically duloxetine or venlafaxine); 2. gabapentin or pregabalin; 3. topical lidocaine for localized pain; 4. opioids or tramadol alone or in combination for acute exacerbations. This group had a stepwise approach to pain management: Step 1 - assessment of patient and investigate causes, comorbidities, including detailed discussion with patient; Step 2 - therapy as above; Step 3 - reassess pain and health-related quality of life, continue therapy if pain is 3/10 or less, consider second- or third-line therapy if unsuccessful and if needed, referral to pain specialist or pain clinic.

Evidence-based guidelines for the treatment of diabetic neuropathic pain, AAN (American Academy of Neurology), AANEM (American Association of Neuromuscular and Electrodiagnostic Medicine), and AAPMR (American Academy of Physical Medicine and Rehabilitation) (3)

This group based their recommendations for the treatment of diabetic neuropathic pain on a literature search of MEDLINE and EMBASE of fully published peer-reviewed articles between 1960 and August 2008. Both pharmacological and nonpharmacological approaches were considered. Among 2234 abstracts used to identify full-length papers, 79 articles were included, excluding case reports and review articles. Based on Class I evidence, pregabalin was established as a Level A Recommendation as effective in lessening the pain of peripheral diabetic neuropathy and

improving quality of life and sleep. Gabapentin and sodium valproate were classified as probably effective and given a Level B Recommendation. A flag concerning the risk of birth defects was placed for sodium valproate. Other agents deemed probably effective (Level B) were: amitriptyline, venlafaxine, duloxetine, dextromethorphan, morphine sulfate, tramadol, oxycodone, capsaicin, isorbide dinitrate, and percutaneous electrical stimulation. Topiramate, desipramine, imipramine, fluoxetine or the combination of nortriptyline and fluphenazine, and alpha lipoic acid had insufficient evidence for or against their use. Oxcarbazepine, lamotrigine, lacosamide, clonidine, pentoxifylline, and mexiletine had evidence against their effectiveness (negative Level B Recommendation).

National Institute of Health and Clinical Excellence (NICE, United Kingdom; from: www.nice.org.uk/guidance/cg96)

This analysis considered 34 forms of pharmacological treatment for neuropathic pain and examined 23,207 studies including 90 randomized controlled clinical trials including economic evidence. The guidelines recommended duloxetine for painful diabetic neuropathy as first-line therapy. If this agent was contraindicated, amitriptyline then pregabalin were the next choices. Third-line treatment considered tramadol alone or in combination with second-line therapies. Topical lidocaine was suggested for localized pain. Duloxetine was thought to be the most cost effective treatment followed by amitriptyline and pregabalin.

Commentary on guidelines

Taken together, these guidelines for the treatment of neuropathic pain provide relatively similar recommendations. The AAN guidelines focus on diabetic neuropathic pain, unlike the others listed. First-line recommendations (or Level A Recommendations) vary because of differences in diabetic and nondiabetic neuropathic pain trials as well as differing criteria for weighting of the evidence (e.g., % study population retention).

Specific agents[1]

Calcium channel α2-δ ligands, gabapentin, and pregabalin

Gabapentin can be initiated in low doses (e.g., 300 mg qhs) and increased to 300 mg tid to a maximum of 3600–4000 mg daily. It does not interfere with the metabolism of other drugs and is nominally nonsedative and nonaddictive. Side-effects are: dizziness, fatigue, and cognitive complaints with initial usage or higher doses, and lower limb edema. These agents are excreted by the kidney (dose reduction in renal failure). Pregabalin can be started at 75 mg qhs, titrated up to 75 mg bid to a maximum of 600 mg daily. The side-effect profile is similar to gabapentin.

Serotonin and norepinephrine reuptake inhibitors (SSRIs and SSNRIs; antidepressants)

Venlafaxine can be initiated at 37.5 mg/day and increased weekly by 37.5 mg/day to a maximum of 225 mg/day. Side-effects are: nausea, dizziness, drowsiness, hyperhidrosis, hypertension, and constipation. Duloxetine can be started at 30 mg daily titrated up to a maximum of 120 mg daily. Side-effects are: risk of hepatotoxicity, nausea, dry mouth, constipation, somnolence, hyperhidrosis, and decreased appetite. Amitriptyline can be started at 10–25 mg qhs once daily then titrated up to 100–150 mg. Side-effects include next day drowsiness, lethargy, dry mouth, constipation, and bladder retention; amitriptyline may help with prominent nocturnal pain; exert caution in patients with cardiac conduction abnormalities or prostatic hypertrophy.

---

[1] Therapeutic agents are only briefly described here and recommendations are listed as suggestions only. Clinicians should be aware that recommended therapy for pain or other disorders may change with time and the regimens and approvals vary with the jurisdiction. All therapeutics should be used only with complete reference to indications, contraindications, adverse effects, and dosage. These suggestions are also not based on specific FDA approval in the United States.

Opioids

Tramadol can be initiated at 37.5 mg po q3–6h, and is often combined with 325 mg of acetaminophen [long-acting preparations starting at a single dose of 100–150 mg daily to a maximum of 300–400 mg daily]; long-acting (controlled-release) oxycodone 10–100 mg can be given divided into twice daily administration [ratio of efficacy to morphine is 1.5 mg oxycodone/1.0 mg morphine]; morphine sulfate is given as 30–60 mg bid of a long-acting preparation (e.g., MS contin) and may be the treatment of choice with severe unremittant pain and severe underlying systemic disease (e.g., renal failure, cardiac disease); side-effects from opioids are as follows: cognitive dysfunction, somnolence, respiratory depression, constipation, pruritus, dizziness, nausea, vomiting, and rebound headache syndrome; risk of addiction, dose escalation, and withdrawal syndrome; questionable risk of suicidal ideation from oxycodone.

Local agents

The 5% lidocaine patch can be used in post-herpetic neuralgia. It is applied to the area of painful skin for 12 h and then removed for the next 12 h. The efficacy may not be potent enough in monotherapy but it can be a useful supplement to systemic treatment and has few side-effects. The 8% capsaicin patch is licensed in Europe for peripheral neuropathic pain excepting that from diabetic neuropathy. It is applied to the painful skin for 30 min after local anesthesia and may provide pain relief for up to 12 weeks. Side-effects may be local reactions and an initial increased burning pain.

References

(1) Attal N, Cruccu G, Haanpaa M, et al. EFNS guidelines on pharmacological treatment of neuropathic pain. *Eur J Neurol* 2006;13:1153–1169.

(2) Dworkin RH, O'Connor AB, Audette J, et al. Recommendations for the pharmacological management of neuropathic pain: an overview and literature update. *Mayo Clin Proc* 2010;85:S3–S14.

(3) Bril V, England J, Franklin GM, et al. Evidence-based guideline: treatment of painful diabetic neuropathy: report of the American Academy of Neurology, the American Association of Neuromuscular and Electrodiagnostic Medicine, and the American Academy of Physical Medicine and Rehabilitation. *Neurology* 2011;76:1758–1765.

Index

acetaminophen
  CIDP 43
  herpes zoster 37, 38
  lumbosacral plexopathy 23

acid-sensing ion channels 8

acroparesthesia 72

alendronate 79

algesic molecules 4–5, 22

allodynia 2, 5, 28
  amyloid-associated polyneuropathy 63
  central post-stroke pain 104, 106
  chronic migraine 115
  CRPS 79
  diabetic polyneuropathy 46
  herpes zoster 39
  sarcoidosis 68
  syringomyelia 101

allopurinol 50

amiloride 50

amitriptyline 137
  amyloid-associated polyneuropathy 63
  anti-MAG polyneuropathy 61
  central post-stroke pain 105
  CIDP 43
  CRPS 77
  diabetic polyneuropathy 46
  migraine 116
  neuralgic amyotrophy 36
  phantom pain 84
  sarcoidosis 68
  vasculitic neuropathy 54, 55, 57

amputations, phantom pain 84–87

amyloid-associated polyneuropathy 62–65
  pain characteristics 64

amyloidosis 43

amyotrophic lateral sclerosis 93–95
  pain characteristics 94–95

analgesic molecules 5

anti-MAG polyneuropathy 59–61
  pain characteristics 60–61

anti-neutrophil cytoplasmic antibodies 54

arachidonic acid 22

arreflexia 42

arthralgia 68

ASIC channels 29

ATP 4

axonal endbulbs 3

azathioprine
  CIDP 41, 43
  vasculitic neuropathy 54, 56

baclofen
  amyotrophic lateral sclerosis 95
  multiple sclerosis 111
  vasculitic neuropathy 57

balance, loss of 50

benserazide 90

beta-endorphin 5

bisphosphonates in CRPS 78, 79

borrelia-associated radiculitis 30–32

botulinum toxin in amyotrophic lateral sclerosis 95

brachial neuritis 34–36

brachial plexus 35
  injury 19

bradykinin 4, 61

brainstem relays 10–11

Brown-Séquard syndrome 96–98

Bruns-Garland syndrome. See lumbosacral plexopathy

burning feet 44, 64, 68

calcitonin 79

calcitonin gene-related peptide 4, 18

calcium channel α2-δ ligands 137

candesartan 50

cannabinoids 5
  multiple sclerosis pain 111

capsaicin 68, 137
  CIDP 43

carbamazepine
  Fabry disease 72
  neuralgic amyotrophy 36
  paroxysmal hemicrania 122
  phantom pain 84
  trigeminal neuralgia 108, 126, 128
  vasculitic neuropathy 54, 55, 57

carpal tunnel release 17, 18

carpal tunnel syndrome 16–18, 45, 70, 104
  pain characteristics 17–18
  risk factors 17

causalgia 18, 77

celecoxib 50
  paroxysmal hemicrania 124

central post-stroke pain 104–106

cerebral ischemia, acute 130–133
  pain characteristics 132–133

cervical radiculopathy 19–22
  pain characteristics 21–22

cesamet 43

chemokines 4, 25

chronic constriction injury 29

chronic inflammatory demyelinating polyneuropathy. See CIDP

CIDP 41–44, 61
  pain characteristics 44

citalopram 77

clodronate 79

cluster headache 118–121
  differential diagnosis 119
  pain characteristics 120–121
  prevalence 119

CMAPs
  amyloid-associated polyneuropathy 62
  CIDP 42
  diabetic polyneuropathy 45
  painful idiopathic polyneuropathy 50

polyneuropathy 59
vasculitic neuropathy 54

codeine
  CIDP 43
  herpes zoster 37
  lumbosacral plexopathy 23
  painful idiopathic polyneuropathy
    51

complex regional pain syndromes 6,
  18, 77–80
  pain characteristics 78–80

compound motor action potentials. *See*
  CMAPs

constipation 23, 30, 32

cortical pain centers 11

corticosteroids
  carpal tunnel syndrome 17
  CRPS 79
  sarcoidosis 68

cranial neuritis 39

CRPS. *See* complex regional pain
  syndrome

cyclooxygenases 4, 22

cyclophosphamide
  CIDP 41
  sarcoidosis 68
  vasculitic neuropathy 55

cyclosporine A
  sarcoidosis 68
  vasculitic neuropathy 55

cytokines 25
  anti-inflammatory 5

dantrolene 95

decompressive surgery 17

deep brain stimulation 91

dexamethasone 120

diabetes mellitus 45

diabetic amyotrophy 23–26

diabetic polyneuropathy 45–48
  experimental studies 46–48
  pain characteristics 46–48

diabetic thoracoabdominal
  radiculopathy 32

diazepam in CIDP 41, 43

diclofenac 36
  phantom pain 84

diltiazem 57

dimenhydrinate 51

dimethylsulfoxide 79

dorsal root ganglia 6–9, 21

doxepine 122

duloxetine 137
  diabetic polyneuropathy 48

dysarthria 93

dysesthesia 109

ectopic impulses 4

edema 62

electromyography 54
  needle. *See* needle electromyography

enzyme replacement therapy in Fabry
  disease 70, 72

erectile dysfunction 23, 45, 62

erythromelalgia 3, 53

Fabry disease 70–72
  pain characteristics 72

familial amyloidotic polyneuropathy
  63

fentanyl 61
  central post-stroke pain 105
  vasculitic neuropathy 55

flupirtine
  central post-stroke pain 104
  paroxysmal hemicrania 122

foot drop 42, 46, 54

gabapentin 50, 137
  amyloid-associated polyneuropathy
    63
  amyotrophic lateral sclerosis 95
  anti-MAG polyneuropathy 60, 61
  Brown-Séquard syndrome 96
  central post-stroke pain 104,
    105
  cervical radiculopathy 19
  CIDP 43
  diabetic polyneuropathy 46, 48
  Fabry disease 72
  herpes zoster 37, 38
  lumbosacral plexopathy 23, 25
  multiple sclerosis 111
  neuralgic amyotrophy 36
  painful idiopathic polyneuropathy
    51
  sarcoidosis 68
  side-effects 48
  vasculitic neuropathy 54, 57

gait abnormalities
  antalgic gait 50
  ataxic gait 54, 55
  lurching gait 41
  steppage gait 62

galanin 5

gliclazide 23

glucocorticosteroids 120

Guillain-Barré syndrome 35, 36, 60

Hargreaves test 46

headache
  cerebral ischemia 130–133
  cluster 118–121
  migraine 113–116
  multiple sclerosis 110
  paroxysmal hemicrania 122–124
  thunderclap 133

hearing loss 70, 71

heat intolerance 70

herpes zoster 37–40
  pain characteristics 39

herpes zoster ophthalmicus 39

histamine 4

Hoffman sign 93

Horner's sign 16, 19

Horner's syndrome 101

hydromorphone
  CIDP 43
  painful idiopathic polyneuropathy
    51

hydromyelia 99

hyperalgesia 5, 7, 48, 63
  central post-stroke pain 104,
    106
  pressure 79
  syringomyelia 101
  thermal 29

hypoesthesia 104

hypohidrosis 70, 71, 72

hyponatremia 54, 55

ICAM-1 22, 26

indomethacin
  mode of action 124
  paroxysmal hemicrania 122, 123

inflammation 6

inflammatory mediators 4

inherited sensitivity to pressure palsy
  43

interleukin-1β 4

interleukin-6 22

intracellular adhesion molecule-1. *See*
  ICAM-1

intracranial pressure 132

intravenous gamma globulin 41, 43

Jannetta operation 108

Kennedy's disease 93

lamotrigine
central post-stroke pain 105
multiple sclerosis 111

lateral femoral cutaneous nerve of the thigh 27

levodopa 90

Lhermitte's sign 94, 108, 109, 110
causes 110

lidocaine 68, 137

losartan 37

lumbar spondylosis 28

lumbosacral plexopathy 23–26, 45
etiology 25
pain characteristics 25

Lyme radiculopathy 30–32
pain characteristics 32

MAG. *See* myelin-associated glycoprotein

mechanosensitivity 28
ion channels involved in 29

meningismus 130

meperidine 43

meralgia paraesthetica 27–29
pain characteristics 28–29

metamizole 104

met-enkephalin 5

methotrexate 68
polymyalgia rheumatica 83

methylprednisolone
CIDP 41
cluster headache 120
trigeminal neuralgia 108

methysergide 116

migraine disability assessment scale (MIDAS) 115

migraine, chronic 113–116
differential diagnosis 115
pain characteristics 115–116
prevalence 115

mirror therapy in phantom pain 86

misoprostol 111, 128

monoclonal gammopathy 59

morphine 61, 137
CIDP 43
diabetic polyneuropathy 46
phantom pain 84
vasculitic neuropathy 57

motor neuron disease 68

multiple sclerosis 108–111
pain characteristics 109–111

muscle cramps 55, 56, 57

muscle weakness
CIDP 41
herpes zoster 37

myelin-associated glycoprotein 60

myotonic dystrophy type 2 74–76
pain characteristics 75–76

nabilone 51

naftidrofuryl 57

needle electromyography
amyotrophic lateral sclerosis 93
diabetic polyneuropathy 45
herpes zoster 39
myotonic dystrophy type 2 74
polymyalgia rheumatica 82

nerve conduction velocity 70

nerve growth factor 4

nervi nervorum 3, 5–6

neuralgic amyotrophy 34–36
pain characteristics 35–36

neurogenic inflammation 5–6

neuromyotonia 57

neuropathic pain 2

neuropathic pain mechanisms 12
algesic molecules 4–5
analgesic molecules 5
brainstem relays 10–11
cortical pain centers 11
dorsal horn of spinal cord 9–10
ectopic impulses 4
nervi nervorum 5–6
sensory dorsal root ganglia 6–9
thalamic 11
Wallerian degeneration 6

Neuropathic Pain Symptom Inventory (NPSI) 32

neuropathy 2

nifedipine 23

nitric oxide 4, 22, 61

nociceptin 5

nociception 3

non-steroidal anti-inflammatory drugs. *See* NSAIDs

norepinephrine reuptake inhibitors 137

nortriptyline
CIDP 43
vasculitic neuropathy 57

novamine sulfone 124

NSAIDs
Brown-Séquard syndrome 96
central post-stroke pain 104
Parkinson's disease 89, 91

obesity 27, 30

omeprazole 50

opioids 48, 137
See also specific drugs

osteoarthritis 27, 50

osteoporosis 55

oxcarbazepine
trigeminal neuralgia 128
vasculitic neuropathy 55, 57

oxycodone 54, 137
central post-stroke pain 104
herpes zoster 38
vasculitic neuropathy 57

oxycontin 61
amyloid-associated polyneuropathy 63
CIDP 43
painful idiopathic polyneuropathy 51

oxygen therapy in cluster headache 119

pain experience 2

painful idiopathic polyneuropathy 50–53
pain characteristics 52–53

pamidronate 79

paresthesiae 2
amyloid-associated polyneuropathy 62, 63
anti-MAG polyneuropathy 60
CIDP 41
lumbosacral plexopathy 23
syringomyelia 100

Parkinson's disease 89–91
pain characteristics 90–91

paroxysmal extreme pain disorder 3, 7, 53

paroxysmal hemicrania 119, 122–124
pain characteristics 124

Parsonage-Turner syndrome. *See* neuralgic amyotrophy

patent foramen ovale 132

periumbilical angioektasia 70, 71

Phalen's sign 16, 17

phantom pain 84–87

phenytoin
Fabry disease 70, 72
vasculitic neuropathy 55

phonophobia 115, 120, 124

photophobia 115, 120, 124

pins and needles 16

plasma exchange 43

polymyalgia rheumatica 82–83
pain characteristics 83

polyneuropathy
amyloid-associated 62–65
anti-MAG 59–61
CIDP 41–44
Fabry disease 70–72
painful idiopathic 50–53

postherpetic neuralgia 39

postural hypotension 62

prednisolone 34
cluster headache 118
CRPS 79

prednisone 43
CIDP 41
cluster headache 120
polymyalgia rheumatica 82, 83

pregabalin 137
amyotrophic lateral sclerosis 95
Brown-Séquard syndrome 96
central post-stroke pain 104, 105
diabetic polyneuropathy 46, 48
herpes zoster 38
Lyme radiculopathy 32
multiple sclerosis 109, 111
neuralgic amyotrophy 36
painful idiopathic polyneuropathy 51
Parkinson's disease 89
sarcoidosis 68
syringomyelia 100
trigeminal neuralgia 128
vasculitic neuropathy 55, 57

pressure palsy, inherited sensitivity to 17

propranolol 116

prostaglandin E2 22

prostaglandins 4

proteinase-activated receptors 4

quantitative sensory testing 53, 70, 72

quinidine 55

quinine 50, 57

Ramsay Hunt syndrome 39

Randall-Selitto test 46

reflex sympathetic dystrophy 6, 18, 77

reflexes 16, 30, 62, 104
ankle 23, 24, 50, 59
biceps 37
brachioradialis 37
plantar 19, 30
quadriceps 23, 24, 27, 28
triceps 19, 21

riluzole 93

Romberg sign 23, 45, 46, 50, 59, 62

ropivacaine 86

sarcoid peripheral neuropathy 66–68
pain characteristics 68

Schwann cells 4, 61

sensory loss
anti-MAG polyneuropathy 59
carpal tunnel syndrome 16, 18
CIDP 41
lumbosacral plexopathy 23
Lyme radiculopathy 30
meralgia paresthetica 27

sensory nerve action potentials. *See* SNAPs

SEPT9 gene mutation 36

serotonin re-uptake inhibitors 137

shoulder pain in neuralgic amyotrophy 34–36

small fiber neuropathy 66, 67

SNAPs
amyloid-associated polyneuropathy 62
CIDP 41
Fabry disease 70
polyneuropathy 59

spasticity 94

spinal cord
compression 21
dorsal horn 9–10
injury 97

spondylosis 21

substance P 4, 18

Sudeck's atrophy 77

sumatriptan
cluster headache 118, 120
migraine 113
paroxysmal hemicrania 124

SUNCT 124

sural nerve biopsy 51, 63

synthroid 37

syringobulbia 100

syringomyelia 99–102
pain characteristics 101–102

tabes dorsalis 3

thalamic syndrome 105, 106

thalamus 11

thunderclap headache 133

Tinel's sign 16, 17, 18, 28

tizanidine 95

topiramate
migraine 113, 116
multiple sclerosis 111
painful idiopathic polyneuropathy 51
trigeminal neuralgia 128

tramadol 31, 137
diabetic polyneuropathy 48
phantom pain 84
vasculitic neuropathy 55

transcutaneous electrical nerve stimulation (TENS)
painful idiopathic polyneuropathy 51
phantom pain 84

transient ischemic attacks 132

transient receptor potential channels 29

transient receptor potential proteins 8

trazodone 50

treatment 135–137
EFNS guidelines 135
evidence-based 136
IASP recommendations 136
NICE guidelines 136
See also specific drugs

tremor 50

tricyclic antidepressants 48
central post-stroke pain 104

trigeminal neuralgia 108, 109, 110, 126–129
pain characteristics 128

trigemino-autonomic cephalalgias 123

trigeminovascular decompression 108

TRPA1 channel 29

TRPV1 channel 29

TRPV4 channel 29

tumor necrosis factor α 4, 26, 61

V30M mutation 64

valproate

migraine 116

trigeminal neuralgia 128

vasculitic neuropathy 54–58

pain characteristics 57

venlafaxine 137

painful idiopathic polyneuropathy 51

verapamil 120

vertigo 130

vitamin B complex 57

Wallerian degeneration 6

Wallerian-like degeneration 6

weight loss 23

white matter lesions 72

zoster radiculitis 37–40

zoster sine herpete 39